LOOK YOUNGER NATURALLY

The ultimate anti-ageing bible

Health&Fitness MAGAZINE

Words Antonia Kanczula
Photography Ian Hooton
Editor Mary Comber
Art editors Claire Punter, Fanni Williams, Holly White
Sub-editors Sheila Reid, Emma Lewis, Margaret Bartlett, Eve Boggenpoel
Models Laura @ MOT, Tess Montgomery @ MOT
Clothing adidas by Stella McCartney (adidas.com); American Apparel
(americanapparel.co.uk); Earth Couture by Kelly Hoppen (earth-couture.com);
Finisterre (finisterreuk.com); Nike (nikestore.com); Pull-in (pull-in.com); Reebok
(reebok.com); Sweaty Betty (sweatybetty.com); Wellicious (wellicious.com)
Still-life photography Julian Velasquez
Recipes Lyndon Gee

Digital production manager Nicky Baker
Bookazine manager Dharmesh Mistry
Operations director Robin Ryan
Bookazine advertising manager Katie Wood
Managing director of advertising Julian Lloyd-Evans
Newstrade director David Barker
Editorial director Pete Muir
Publishing director Richard Downey
Managing director James Burnay
Chief operating officer Brett Reynolds
Group financial director Ian Leggett
Chief executive officer James Tye
Chairman Felix Dennis

MAG**BOOK**

Look Younger Naturally ISBN 1-907779-26-4

To license this product please contact Hannah Heagney on +44 (0) 20 7907 6134 or e-mail hannah_heagney@dennis.co.uk

DIET PROTEIN™

A PROTEIN BASED DIET SHAKE BRINGING YOU THE LATEST ADVANCES IN NUTRACEUTICALS TO HELP CONTROL BODY WEIGHT AND FAT LEVELS.

PERFORMANCE

Diet Protein™ contains unique bioactive peptides & 100% RDA of calcium
Diet Protein™ uses a unique ratio of purified micellar casein and whey protein to provide an unrivalled source of protein that contains bioactive peptides that may help curb appetite, boost glutathionine levels (antioxidants), promote healthy intestinal flora and provide essential amino acids for recovery from strenuous exercise. In addition to providing an extremely high quality source of protein, Diet Protein™ also provides natural dairy calcium which is scientifically proven to assist in accelerating fat and weight loss by up to 25%*.

Diet Protein™ contains Clarinol™ CLA, a safe, natural, research proven diet aid
One daily serving of Diet Protein™ provides 3.2g of Clarinol™. Lipid Nutrition who produce Clarinol™ have patents under licence that are filed with the FDA that legally allow them to make a series of claims, the following of which clearly illustrate its effectiveness;

Clarinol™ reduces the amount of body fat. Clarinol™ reduces weight gain. Clarinol™ reduces the side effects from a low calorie diet.

Recently completed research** has confirmed that 3.2g of Clarinol™, the exact same as found in Diet Protein™, not only easily helped reduce body fat,
but that it did so in specific areas of the body where fat loss is most desired without extra dieting or exercise efforts.
The results of the six month clinical trial showed that the reduction in fat mass primarily occurs in the abdomen and particularly in women, the legs.

Whilst other diet shakes might contain CLA it is often in smaller amounts. Research proves that you need to take 3.2g or more of CLA to see the best results.

HEALTH

Diet Protein™ provides additional nutraceutical support
Each serving of Diet Protein™ is packed with additional diet support. Green tea extract is added for its long standing reputation for aiding dieters, whilst friendly LactoSpore® probiotic bacteria provide intestinal support.

Diet Protein™ has a very low glycemic index (GI)
Diet Protein™ contains no added sugar or maltodextrin. It's perfect for dieters wanting to restrict their carbohydrate content.

Amazing taste
Diet Protein™ comes in a variety of mouthwatering flavours, all of which have been optimized by our taste testing panel to ensure that they are the best tasting diet shakes on the market.

Made to the highest standards
Diet Protein™ is made by Reflex Nutrition in the UK in accordance with ISO9001 procedures to ensure the highest levels of quality control. Each batch is then tested in our R&D lab for its protein content to ensure it meets our industry leading claims. It's also made with 100% Green Energy.

18 Servings per bag
Available in chocolate, strawberry and banoffee flavours

PERFORMANCE & HEALTH WITHIN

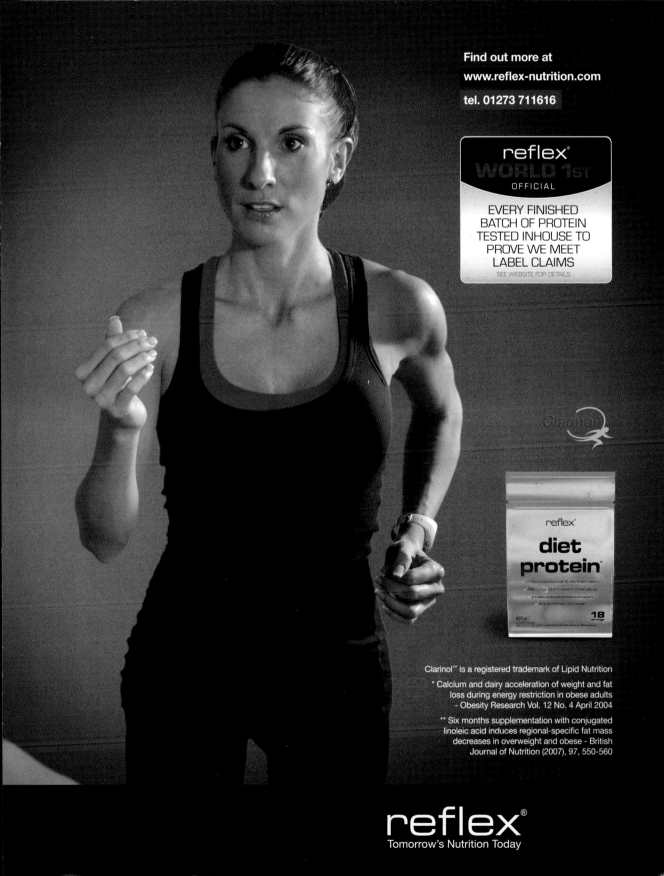

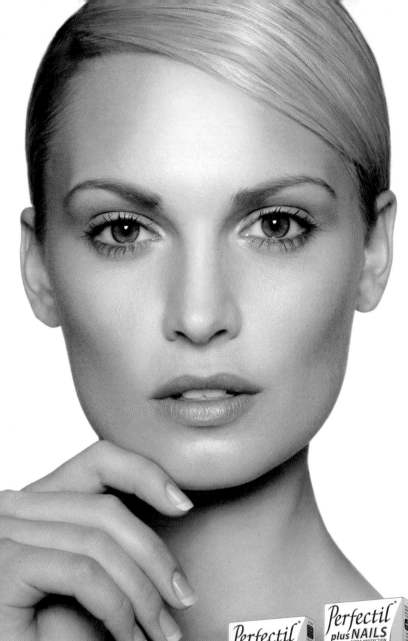

essential beauty for
skin, hair & nails
from within

Advance your beauty regime with *Perfectil*, the UK's No. 1 original Triple-Active™ formula for **skin**, **hair** and **nails**.

Perfectil® Plus Skin provides extra skin protection, while new *Perfectil® Plus Nails* helps support healthy nail growth.

For the ultimate TimeDefy™ formula, there's *Perfectil® Platinum*.

Each replaces your usual multivitamin, so *Perfectil®* can fit easily with your daily routine.

Perfectil® – because true radiance starts from within.

UK's **No 1** SKIN, HAIR & NAILS FORMULA

TalkPerfection.com
Britain's true beauty forum

Don't miss out! Visit Talk Perfection, Britain's one-stop beauty forum.
· Amazing product give aways
· Free trials & new beauty products
· Expert answers to <u>your</u> questions
· Beauty news before it happens

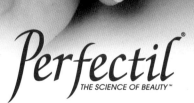

Perfectil®
THE SCIENCE OF BEAUTY™

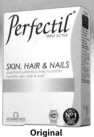

Original
for Skin, Hair & Nails

Extra Nail Protection

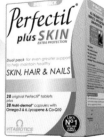

Extra Skin Protection

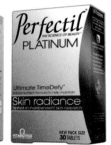

Ultimate TimeDefy™
in 60s or new 30s pack

VITABIOTICS

THE QUEEN'S AWARDS FOR ENTERPRISE 2008

Britain's leading supplements
for specific life stages

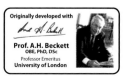

Originally developed with

Prof. A.H. Beckett
OBE, PhD, DSc
Professor Emeritus
University of London

From **Boots**, Superdrug, Holland & Barrett, Lloydspharmacy, supermarkets, chemists, Harrods, GNC, health stores & **perfectil.com**

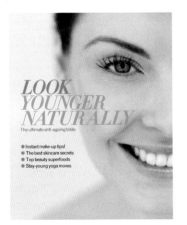

LOOK YOUNGER NATURALLY

The ultimate anti-ageing bible

● Instant make-up tips!
● The best skincare secrets
● Top beauty superfoods
● Stay-young yoga moves

CONTENTS

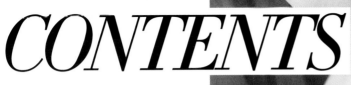

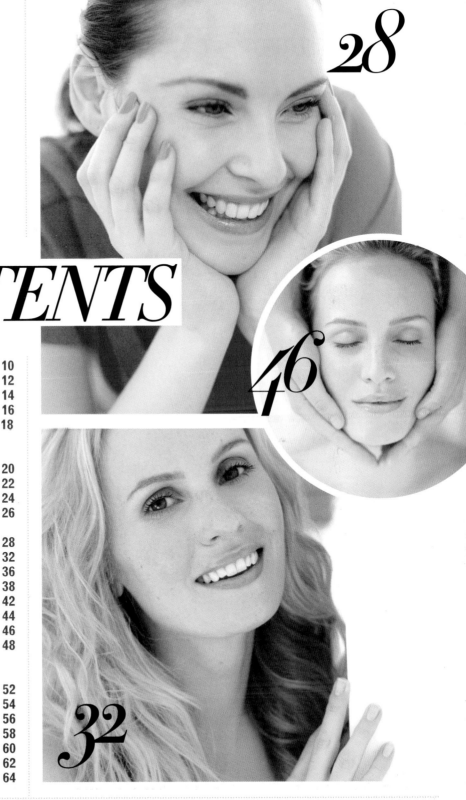

28

46

32

CONTENTS

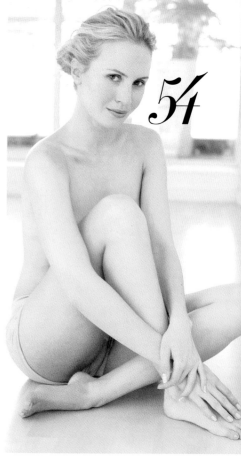

54

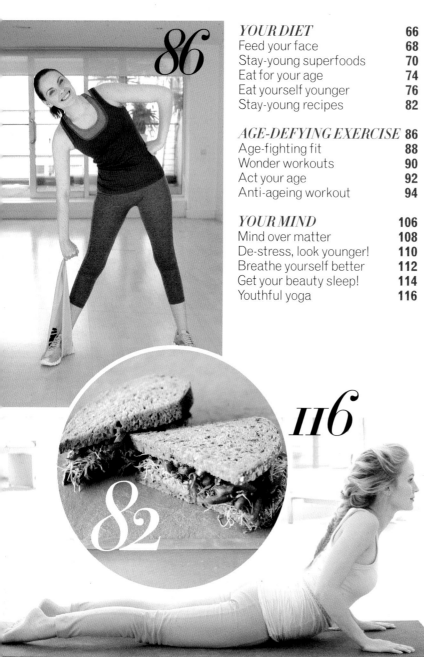

86

116

82

If you'd like more information on the products and services mentioned throughout the book, see the stockists' directory on page 126.

START YOUR DAY WITH
SOLGAR WHEY

Did you know that whey protein has many health benefits?
weight management • ageing • bone health

BANANA BEAUTY BOOST - A NUTRITIOUS RECIPE FOR YOU

This sweet nutty smoothie contains essential fats, protein, vitamin E, magnesium, fibre and potassium – nutrients that promote healthy skin, nails and hair. Served thick, this makes a great breakfast.

Serves 1
■ Calories 419 ■ Fat 13.9g ■ Saturated fat 1.2g ■ Carbohydrates 46.6g ■ Fibre 9.5g ■ Protein 28g

• 1 banana (chopped and frozen – optional)
• ½ tbsp almond butter
• 1 scoop Solgar *Whey to Go® Protein Powder* –Vanilla flavour
• 1 tsp Solgar *Omega Advanced Blend 2:1:1*
• ½ tbsp ground flaxseeds
• 1 tbsp oatbran / oats / wheatgerm (optional)
• Water – enough to create the desired consistency

Blend all ingredients together and serve immediately

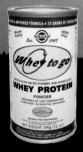
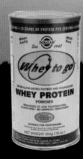
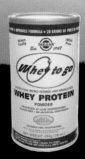

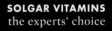
SOLGAR VITAMINS
the experts' choice

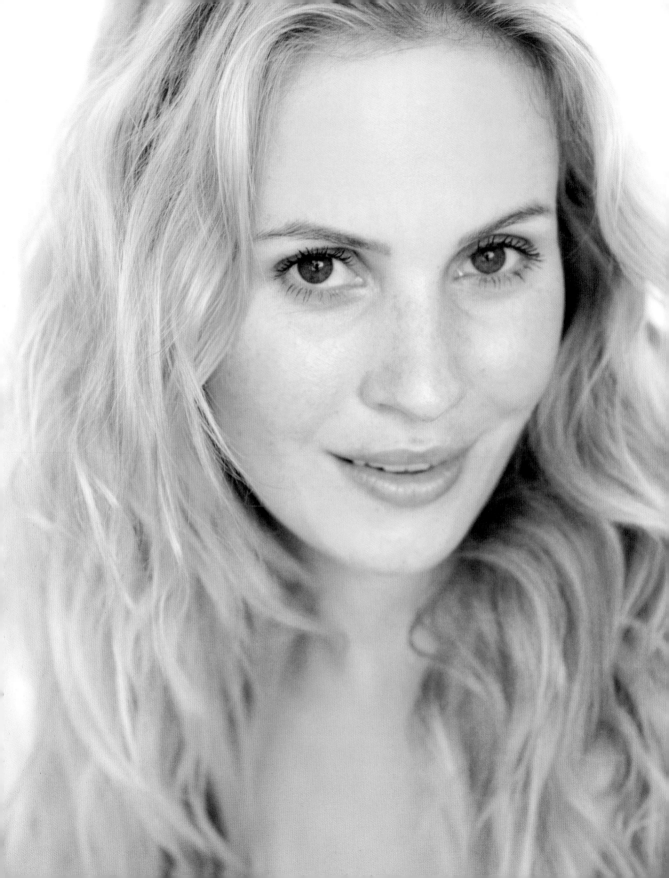

Welcome!

Looking and staying youthful is about so much more than anti-ageing creams. In this book you'll find easy, natural ways to feel and look your best, at every stage of your life

Back in our teens, we'd do anything to appear older and more mature. Then, in a rapid about-turn, we reach adulthood and hanker after the supple skin and litheness of our formative years.

The good news is, you don't have to resort to cosmetic surgery to stay looking your best. There are plenty of effective, natural steps you can take every day. Scientific research is increasingly proving that your genetic make-up is not the only determinant of how quickly – or slowly – you age. Your diet, exercise, lifestyle habits and skincare regime all play a key role in how youthful you look and feel. The way you eat, breathe, sleep – and even think – can accelerate or slow down the ageing process. By making some simple lifestyle changes, you can easily look 10 years younger – and feel more vital and energised!

This book shows you the latest, natural ways to turn back the clock. You'll find everything from anti-ageing skincare secrets to stay-young foods and the best exercise to keep you toned, strong and flexible.

YOUR NATURAL ANTI-AGEING PLAN
Staying young isn't just about slathering the latest must-have cream onto your face. In this book, we look at ageing inside and out. We'll explain how the ageing process works, and reveal ways to reduce the key age accelerators to keep all of your body, including your heart, eyes, fertility, brain and, of course, your skin, youthful – without the aid of cosmetic surgery. Find out how to eat yourself younger with anti-ageing superfoods, stretch and breathe your way to a more youthful body with an exercise plan, and use easy make-up and haircare tricks to erase years from your appearance.

WHATEVER YOUR LIFE STAGE
It's easy to associate ageing with fine lines and the odd grey hair and forget the positive benefits of being older – things that concerned you in your youth seem less important as you become more confident in yourself. And with each decade, new challenges and the skills you develop to meet them all go towards making you who you are.

So rather than thinking of age-proofing your body

> *Simple changes to your diet and daily regimes can naturally turn back your body clock*

as a self-improvement regime, see it as looking after yourself as you age. It won't just make you look and feel younger and boost your health, it can be fun too – in fact, we'll be praising the benefits of shopping, sex, laughter, wine and chocolate! Of course, there's no magic pill, but taking a proactive approach to your health and wellbeing during each stage of your life will ensure you look and feel your best, whatever your age. So whether you're in your 20s, 30s, 40s or beyond, this book will give you all the age-specific tips you need to see the changes you want.

7 *LOOK YOUNGER SECRETS*

The ultimate ways to stay youthful – from head to toe

NOURISH

A healthy, nutrient-rich diet keeps your body young inside – and outside. Take a look at our chapter on diet and skin, from page 66.

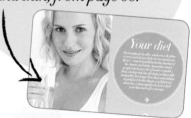

EXERCISE

Nothing beats the post-exercise glow – it's the physical expression of a dynamic circulation. Read our chapter on exercise, starting on page 86.

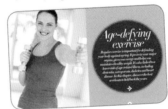

BREATHE

Your skin relies on a ready supply of oxygen and nutrients, so healthy breathing techniques are vital for radiant skin. Turn to page 112 for more details.

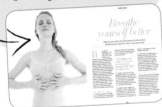

HYDRATE

Drinking water and regular moisturising will keep your skin plump and dewy. Get the lowdown on page 68.

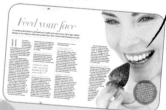

REST

It's not called beauty sleep for nothing, you know – while you snooze, your body repairs and renews itself. Go to page 114 to discover how you can sleep more soundly.

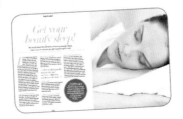

PROTECT

Sun damage is the primary cause of premature wrinkles. For tips on how to protect yourself while still reaping the sun's benefits, turn to page 44.

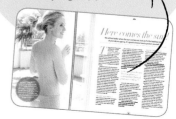

CLEANSE

Your skin is constantly renewing, and cleansing gives it a helping hand by removing dead cells. Find out more on page 24.

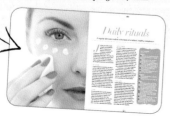

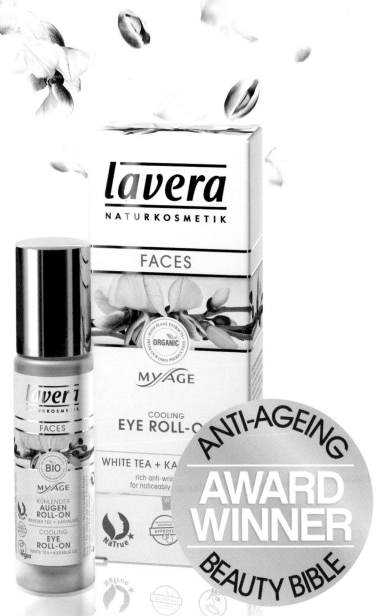

lavera
NATURAL COSMETICS

" eye area was clearer, less puffy and incredibly refreshed - felt fantastic"

· ·

"...the light gel soaks in easily, gives a firming effect; very impressive..."

www.lavera.co.uk

100% natural anti-ageing skin care

no animal testing · no parabens · no SLS/SLES · no petrochemicals

lavera's MY AGE range offers exceptional anti-ageing face care using the powerful active organic ingredients of white tea and karanja oil.

The Cooling Eye Roll-On is a must have to relieve tired and dull looking eyes.

Available in selected health food stores and other outlets or buy online at www.lavera.co.uk

 www.facebook.com/laveranaturalskincare    www.twitter.com/laverauk   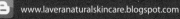 www.laveranaturalskincare.blogspot.com

All change

It happens so subtly, you won't even realise it's going on.
Here's our guide to how your body alters over the decades

Believe it or not, your body starts to age from the physical peak of puberty. And we're not just talking about skin; everything from your bone density to muscle mass starts to wane. Happily, as we'll go on to explain later in the book, there's plenty you can do to slow the speed of change!

After the hormonal ups and downs of your teens, your skin comes into its own in your 20s. New cells are replicating at an enviable pace, so your complexion should be plump and radiant. Towards the end of the decade, fine lines may start to appear on your forehead and around your eyes, particularly if you haven't been taking care of yourself.

This is likely to be your most carefree decade, but skipping sleep and meals and consuming far too much alcohol can deplete your body.

Your bone density is at its peak in your early 20s, as is your natural aerobic fitness and the amount of lean, metabolism-revving muscle you carry. Even your brain power peaks at 22. Capitalise on the natural advantages of your age and you'll build sound foundations for the future.

ANTI-AGEING ADVICE: Now's the time to start a regular and sustained exercise programme to set yourself in good stead and build up credits for the decades to come.

> **In your 20s, new cells are replicating at an enviable pace, so your complexion should be plump and radiant**

The natural decline in fitness that started in your 20s may manifest itself now in slight weight gain. The ageing process will also show – albeit faintly – on your face. Fine lines will become more evident, your pores may enlarge and radiance decline. You may notice your first grey hairs.

No part of your body is immune to small changes – you may feel a slight stiffness in your muscles and joints and they could be more prone to injury; your breasts will be less full and by the time you're 35, your fertility is half what it was at 25. That's not to say you should think of slowing down – quite the contrary!

ANTI-AGEING ADVICE: You body isn't as resilient as in your 20s, so eat a balanced healthy diet and keep your weight at a healthy level.

The lines of your 30s may become more pronounced wrinkles and you may notice your skin becoming drier, as your body enters the perimenopause – the precursor of the menopause, when you still have periods but experience menopause symptoms, such as hot flushes. As levels of the female hormone oestrogen decline, fat will naturally settle on your abdomen and you'll find it harder to shed the pounds.

Other changes synonymous with ageing may begin now – for instance, your eyesight and hearing won't be quite as sharp as they once were. Your heart isn't as youthful either – as the decade progresses, it has to work harder to pump blood around your body and your blood vessels lose elasticity.

ANTI-AGEING ADVICE: Become breast aware – incidence of breast cancer increases sharply during your 40s and 50s. Go to www.nhs.uk to find out how to check your breasts.

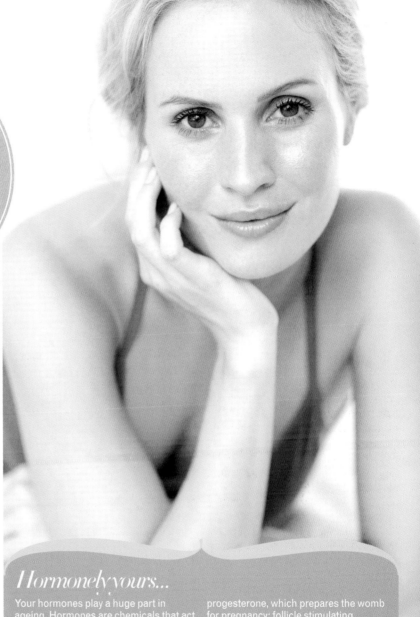

50s plus

Most women enter the menopause in their early 50s. The menopause can affect your body in many ways.

Physically, the drop in oestrogen raises your risk of low bone density, heart disease and breast cancer. Your skin's hydration levels also dwindle, so it's more prone to sensitivity. And the production of collagen, a protein in the skin responsible for its strength and elasticity, slows down, increasing wrinkles.

If you don't do anything to delay it, other signs of ageing include stiffened joints, hair loss, more fat around the tummy and impaired memory. Your digestive system will be slowing down, making you more prone to constipation, and your senses of taste and smell will decline gradually. Because of wear and tear, and a drop in saliva levels, your teeth and gums will also be susceptible.

In your 60s, muscle tissue loss accelerates and, as the cushioning discs between the vertebrae of your spine lose plumpness and depth, your height will also gradually decrease.

ANTI-AGEING ADVICE: Heart disease is your biggest health risk, so eat healthily, exercise regularly and keep cholesterol and blood pressure in check – ask your GP for tests.

Hormonely yours...

Your hormones play a huge part in ageing. Hormones are chemicals that act as messengers between two parts of the body. They influence countless bodily processes, including your metabolism and body clock. There are various hormone 'factories' in your body – for instance, your pancreas produces insulin – and they slow down as you age.

Your reproductive system relies on complex hormonal activity. The key players are oestrogen, which is involved in the release of eggs from the ovaries; progesterone, which prepares the womb for pregnancy; follicle stimulating hormone and luteinizing hormone.

At the menopause – between the ages of 45 and 55 – levels of oestrogen and progesterone plummet and the typical signs of ageing appear. Your skin's elasticity is reduced, your joints may begin to ache and your hair thins. You're also at increased risk of breast cancer, heart disease and osteoporosis. But, as we go on to explain, you can future-proof your body with a healthy lifestyle.

What's ageing you?

Whether or not you look older or younger than your calendar age doesn't just depend on your genes. A cocktail of factors determine how fast you age

The physical signs of ageing may be inevitable, but the pace at which they occur isn't. It's down to a mix of biological 'intrinsic' programming and external or 'extrinsic' factors. And the good news is, a huge body of scientific research highlights just how much control we have over the process. Research from the University of Gothenburg in Sweden has shown that we don't purely 'inherit' longevity – it's the sum total of our lifestyle habits. Meanwhile, a large study by the Public Library of Science Medicine in the UK has established that simple lifestyle changes, such as regular exercise, low alcohol intake and not smoking, can add up to 14 years to your life. Here are the main age-accelerators to beware of.

SEDENTARY LIFESTYLE

Exercise, or rather a lack of it, is one of the most powerful factors contributing to ageing – internally and externally. Staying active helps prevent many conditions and illnesses associated with old age, including heart disease, dementia and osteoporosis. It keeps you mobile for longer and, by boosting your circulation,

makes your skin radiant. But, crucially, exercise also works at a cellular level and, as a result, strengthens your skeleton, improves your digestion and enlarges your heart. A study at King's College, London, and the National Institute on Ageing, Maryland in the US, found a couch potato lifestyle can biologically age you by up to 10 years by shortening chain-like structures called telomeres, which work to protect DNA.

> ❝ *Regular exercise, low alcohol intake and not smoking can add 14 years to your life* ❞

POOR DIET

Eating healthily is crucial for maintaining a healthy weight and preventing age-related diseases, and research shows it will also keep your skin looking youthful too. Choosing the right kind of foods – namely antioxidant-rich fruit and vegetables – can counteract the ageing effects of pesky free radicals (see box for the lowdown on these damaging

scavengers). Drinking plenty of water and eating healthy fats, such as plant oils, are essential for keeping your complexion hydrated and plump. In contrast, an excess of sugary, processed foods can accelerate the breakdown of collagen and elastin fibres, which act as your skin's scaffolding. Eating too much saturated animal fat can overburden your heart and your liver, resulting in a dull and lifeless complexion.

SMOKING

There's no part of your body that isn't affected by smoking. It's detrimental to skin; not only does it decrease oxygen supply so your complexion appears dull and dehydrated, it also generates free radicals and causes those characteristic 'inhale' wrinkles around the mouth. It's said that regular smokers will eventually look 10 to 20 years older than their natural age, and no area of skin is left unsullied, according to experts at the University of Michigan in the US. Inside your body, smoking interferes with the renewal of bones, reducing their density, contributes to the furring of the arteries – a process called atherosclerosis –

damages your lungs and significantly increases the likelihood of oral health problems, such as tooth loss.

SUN

In many ways a blast of sunshine is positively life-enhancing; it flushes your body with vitamin D, which is vital for a healthy immune system, balanced mood and strong bones. And, of course, aesthetically, sun-kissed skin has a natural, healthy glow. However, too much can be a bad thing. As well as upping your risk of skin cancer, sun exposure is recognised as one of most potent complexion-agers, causing, according to dermatologists, a whopping 80 per cent of age-related skin damage. It can contribute to age spots, wrinkles, pigmentation and loss of elasticity. Plus, it ages your hair and eyes. Find out how you can protect yourself, without compromising your wider health, on page 44.

STRESS

Stress used to be merely seen as a state of mind. Now, there's increasing evidence that chronic and prolonged episodes can compromise your health and age your body. Research shows it can disrupt sleep, dampen your immune system, contribute to raised blood pressure, and result in weight gain – which are all ageing. And don't forget that it can also directly contribute to the physical signs of ageing – all that frowning can lead to permanent lines on your forehead! Researchers at Case Western Reserve University in Cleveland, Ohio in the US who studied identical twins, who should age at a similar rate, found that a divorced twin looked almost two years older than their sibling who was single or married. The scientists suggest it was the sustained periods of stress that the divorced twins had been through that was one of the biggest factors in how much faster they aged. And your hair can suffer too – anxiety can thin and accelerate the greying process. We explore the issue of stress further on page 114.

ALCOHOL

An occasional tipple won't do you any harm – in fact various studies, including a recent one on heart disease, published in the *British Medical Journal*, show that moderate drinking is beneficial. However, excess long-term consumption contributes to liver disease, heart problems, weakened bones and has been highlighted as a risk factor in breast cancer. And it's bad for your skin too. Alcohol can dehydrate your complexion, damage elastin and collagen, cause sensitivity and result in broken veins and a ruddy hue.

POLLUTION

On a day-to-day basis, we're bombarded by an array of polluting particles – from paint fumes to chemical air-fresheners to the ultra-fine dust from photocopiers and toxic car exhaust emissions. Our lungs are, without doubt, affected – but so, too, is our skin. According to a recent study conducted at Leibniz Research Institute for Environmental Medicine in Dusseldorf in Germany, the higher the concentration of traffic-related airborne particles, the greater the likelihood of extrinsic skin ageing, particularly pigment spots on the forehead and cheeks.

Free radicals explained

WHAT ARE THEY?

Free radicals are atoms or groups of atoms in our bodies that have electrons missing, so they become highly chemically reactive. To redress their electron imbalance, these scavengers 'steal' electrons from other molecules in your body and, by altering their chemical structure, cause damage to cells, protein and DNA. This can result in increased signs of ageing, as well as contribute to degenerative diseases, such as cancer.

WHAT TRIGGERS THEM?

Free radicals are created in response to your body's interaction with oxygen, and are caused by natural biological processes such as breathing, as well as external pollutants such as toxins and tobacco smoke.

HOW TO COMBAT THEM:

To prevent cellular damage (oxidative stress), increase your intake of antioxidants. Available in fresh fruit and veg, they mop up and neutralise dangerous free radicals and are central to your anti-ageing armour.
Turn to page 66 to learn more.

What's your real age?

Take this fun quiz to find out if your chronological age matches up with your body

This quiz will help highlight the factors that may be prematurely ageing you, so you can adjust your lifestyle accordingly. For each question, use the following scoring system, unless stated.

○ Yes, always – **1 point**
○ Sometimes – **0.5 point**
○ Frankly, no – **0 point**

1. Research shows exercise is good for your heart, bones and brain – and reduces the risk of chronic illnesses. Aerobic exercise, such as swimming, walking and cycling, keeps your heart and lungs youthful.
Do you exercise aerobically every day?

2. We lose muscle mass as we age, which contributes to weight gain and decreased mobility.
Does your weekly workout include resistance exercise, such as weight training?

3. Weight-bearing exercise is vital for healthy bones and includes any activity, such as running, walking or tennis, where your body impacts with the ground.
a) Do your bones get a workout most days?
b) Are you a healthy weight i.e. neither under or overweight?

4. A healthy diet is crucial for keeping your mind and body young. Fresh fruit and veg is bursting with antioxidants and nutrients.
a) Do you get at least five a day?
b) Do you avoid sugar, salt and processed foods?
c) Do you minimise your intake of saturated animal fats and prioritise healthy plant oils?
d) Do you drink plenty of water?

5. Research shows stress speeds up cell ageing.
Do you generally avoid stress and can you cope with stressful situations?

6. Sun exposure causes premature skin ageing and damages your eyes.
Do you take precautions to limit the effects of the sun on your body?
○ Yes, always – **2 points**
○ Sometimes – **1 point**
○ Frankly, no – **0 points**

7. Smoking is damaging for your body, including skin, bones, heart and eyes.
Are you a non-smoker?
○ Yes – **2 points**
○ I like the occasional cigarette and/or I'm regularly exposed to cigarette smoke – **1 point**
○ No, I'm a regular smoker – **0 points**

8. Excess alcohol damages the liver, heart, your fertility, digestion and bones.

Do you stick to the Government's daily recommended allowance of two to three units a day, or are you teetotal?
Yes, always – **2 points**
Sometimes – **1 point**
Frankly, no – **0 points**

9. Studies show lack of sleep raises inflammatory markers which can contribute to premature ageing.
Do you get at least six to eight hours of quality sleep a night?

What your results mean...

a) 12 to 16 points
You're holding back the years, as far as is humanly possible – keep it up!

b) 8 to 11 points
Overall, your outlook is positive, but try to make a couple of healthy changes.

c) 0 to 7 points
Don't leave the ageing process to fate and your DNA – make some simple changes to your lifestyle.

Look Younger Naturally

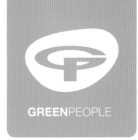

GREENPEOPLE

Green People are pioneers in organic and fairly traded skincare. With 60% of what is put on skin getting absorbed into the bloodstream, simply choosing natural ingredients will make a positive difference to the way you look and feel!

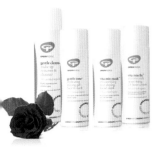

Award-winning and fairly traded

Our skin care range uses the highest quality certified organic ingredients, chosen to nourish and soothe the most sensitive skin. Look younger naturally by switching to organic skincare that is highly effective with natural formulations combining antioxidants and anti-ageing ingredients for wrinkle reduction. High in actives, Omega-3&6, Organic plant extracts and Rosehip Oil to keep skin looking younger and radiant.

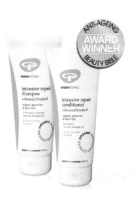

Gorgeous, clean shiny hair!

Is your hair is coloured, flat and lifeless or your scalp itchy and sensitive Green People has the solution. Shampoos with the mildest cleansing and foaming agents derived from pure plant oils. Try Intensive Repair Shampoo and Conditioner with nourishing organic Aloe vera, Green tea and B vitamins to strengthen damaged hair.

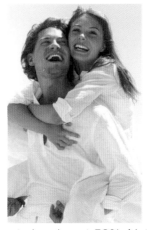

Faster natural sun protection

Tan and protect your skin with broad spectrum UVA & UVB and natural antioxidants – all in one! Our popular Sun Lotion SFP15 contains an extract from the carob tree which naturally stimulates melanin; speeding up the tanning process by 25% and reducing the tan-fading rate by almost 50%. Natural antioxidants and skin vitamins help support the skin's immune system to help avoid premature ageing. Suitable for sensitive skin and prickly heat.

Are you using enough?

As a rough guide, an adult will need 25-30 grams of sun lotion **about a shot glass full** to give the claimed protection over the whole body.

 @GreenPeopleUK

 GreenPeopleOrganic

No Nasties...

Sodium Lauryl/Laureth Sulphate, Parabens, Lanolin, Phthalates, Propylene Glycol, Alcohol (Ethyl Alcohol, Ethanol), Harsh Foaming Agents, Petrochemicals, DEA, TEA or PEGs

FREE Catalogue & trial sachet

www.greenpeople.co.uk
01403 740 350

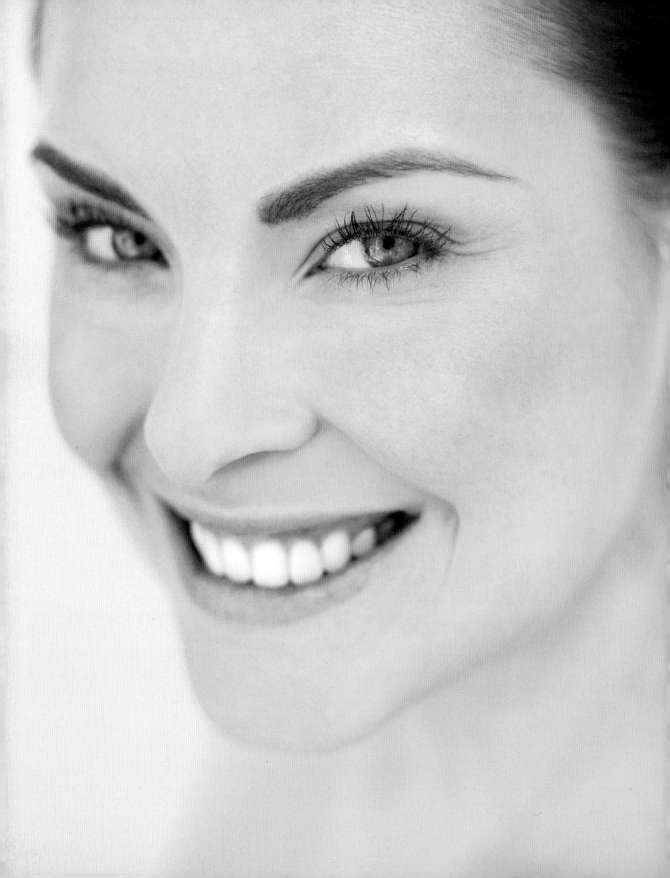

Your skin

Plump and radiant skin is synonymous with youth . But a holistic approach to holding back the years doesn't just entail a dedicated cleanse, tone, moisturise regime – a healthy lifestyle also benefits your skin. To keep your complexion tip-top it helps if you understand your skin, so we're going back to basics in this chapter. Discover more about the function of your skin and how to target key ageing factors. Spritz, pout, dab and massage your way to younger skin... naturally.

Spotlight on your skin

Your skin isn't just a covering for your bones, it's also a complex organ. Understand how it functions and you can learn to take better care of it

Accounting for about 16 per cent of your body weight, you have around two square metres of skin. And it's more than a barrier against the environment. As well as protecting you from harmful UV rays, infection and chemicals, it also regulates your temperature through processes such as sweating, and houses a network of nerves that can detect pain, temperature, pressure, textures, vibration and itches. Your skin also produces vitamin D, which is essential for the growth and maintenance of your bones as well as other important body functions. It's also an underrated mode of communication – your skin can visually express a complex range of emotions by blushing and sweating.

EPIDERMIS
This outer barrier layer of your skin consists of four sub-layers – five on your palms and soles of your feet. It's made mostly of cells called keratinocytes, which produce a protein keratin, the same substance that forms your nails and hair. For something so tough, it's incredibly thin – about 1mm over most of your body. The epidermis is in a constant bottom-upwards process of renewal, which normally takes around 26 to 42 days, but this slows down as you age and dead cells can linger on the surface, leaving skin looking less radiant.

DERMIS
Lying beneath the epidermis and about four times thicker, the dermis comprises

> 66 *Skin houses nerves that detect pain, temperature, pressure, textures, vibration and itches* 99

the papillary layer, nearest the epidermis, and the deeper reticular layer. It contains elements that contribute to your skin's function, including hair follicles, nerve endings, oil glands, blood vessels and sweat glands. The dermis is made up of two proteins, collagen and elastin, which are your skin's scaffolding and decrease with age, plus natural oils and water. Your complexion is also repaired by cells originating in the dermis, such as fibroblasts, which assist with wound repair.

SUBCUTANEOUS LAYER
This fatty layer acts as insulation and its depth varies from person to person. It's involved in synthesising vitamin D, and the blood vessels that fan out into the dermis come from here.

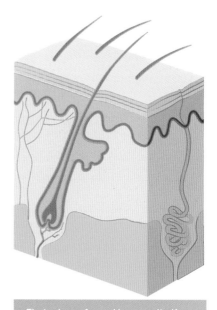

The top layer of your skin renews itself every 26 to 42 days, gradually slowing down as you age.

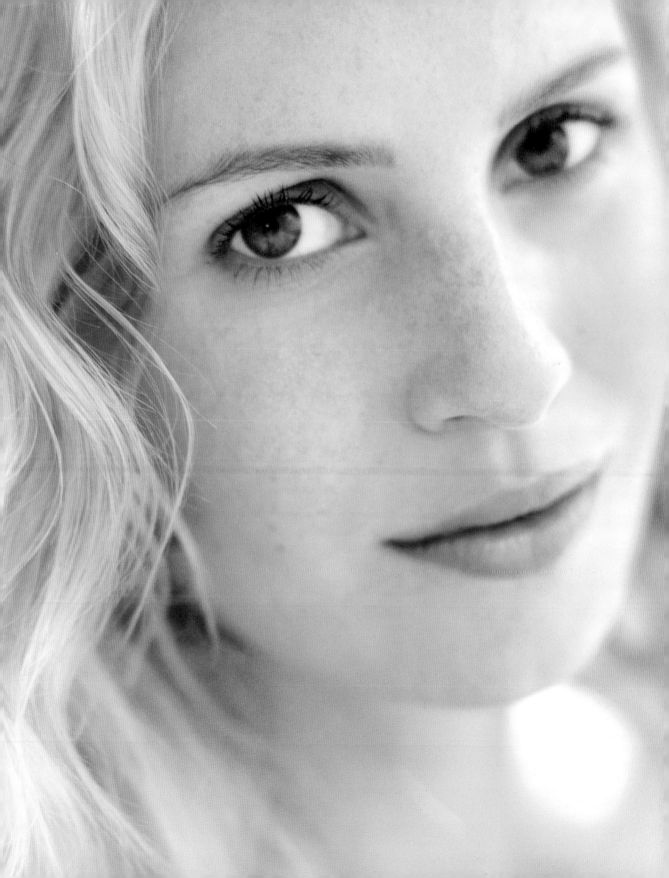

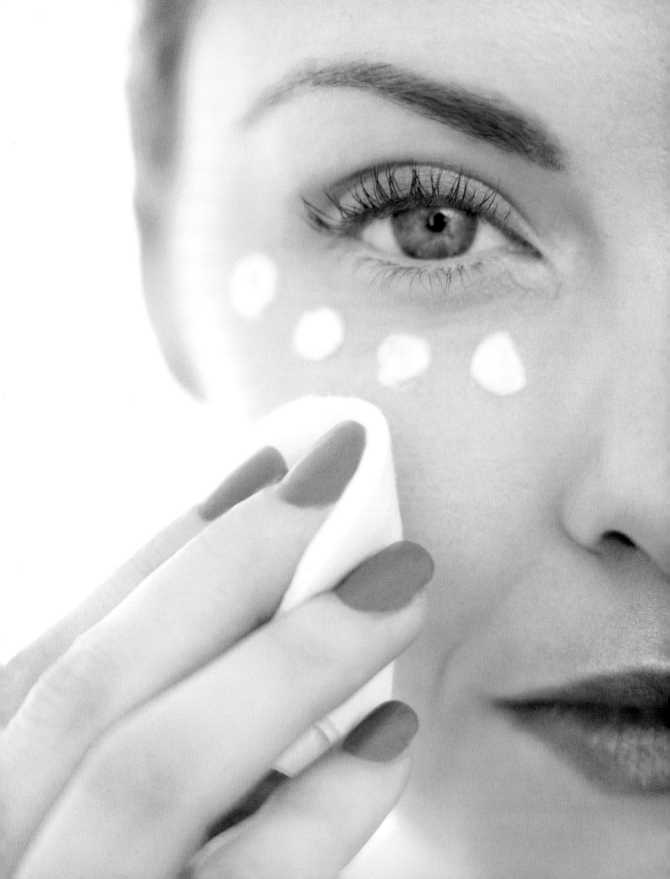

Daily rituals

A regular skincare routine is the basis of a radiant, healthy complexion

Just as your body needs a regular and sustained fitness programme to stay trim and toned, your complexion demands a dedicated approach too. And irrespective of your age or skin type, the fundamentals of skincare are the same. Your skin is a complex and delicate organ, but the principles of caring for it are straightforward and common-sense.

CLEANSE

A good cleanse is essential, not only to remove make-up residue, dirt and grime, but also to shift dead cells and sebum so your skin is left clearer. Apply your cleanser to dry skin, using a light, circular massage technique to bring fresh blood to the skin surface and reduce puffiness. It's tempting to go for products with a lathering quality so your face is squeaky clean, but these tend to be harsh on your skin. Try nourishing, cream cleansers to keep your skin hydrated and prevent sensitivity. Soaps are most definitely out.

TONE

It's not essential, but a gentle sweep of toner across your face can help remove those last few traces of cleanser, and refresh and hydrate your skin. Give alcohol-based products the cold shoulder – it's best go for nutrient-rich products with natural skin benefits, such as aloe vera, cucumber, calendula and rosewater.

MOISTURISE

Your skin contains a natural lipid barrier to protect it against the elements and invaders, such as pollution and dirt. By applying a moisturiser, you're enhancing the strength of your skin's innate shield, and preserving the hydration levels in its deep layers. Choose a protective SPF day cream and an intensive moisturiser or face oil at night. Even if you think your skin is oily, moisturising is essential – use lighter products based on plant oils, so your complexion doesn't get congested.

A moisturiser or foundation with a broad-spectrum SPF15 protection, even on cloudy days, will help prevent UV damage. Added antioxidants are a bonus too. Don't forget to apply to your lips and neck too. Use a stronger sunscreen if you're spending lots of time outside.

EXFOLIATE

Gentle exfoliation will speed up your skin's cellular turnover – but we don't mean abrasive, grainy products. They're a bad idea for sensitive and mature skins. Using a soft muslin cloth is ideal or, for a thorough, occasional exfoliation, choose products that contain alpha hydroxy acids (AHAs), chemical compounds found in citric fruits and cane sugar which act as a natural exfoliant. Or pick products containing fine jojoba beads. How often you use them depends on skin type, but start with once or twice a week. If your skin still appears dull, or flaky, use more regularly.

24/7 care

Morning
- Give your face a quick rinse with a facial wash, if needed, and pat skin gently dry.
- Sweep a soft cotton wool ball loaded with toner across your complexion in an upwards direction.
- Moisturise, ideally with a product that contains reflective sunscreen, in a gentle sweeping upwards motion.
- Apply your eye cream with a gentle, patting action.
- Use an instant radiance serum or balm to restore perkiness.

Daytime
- Spritz your skin with a hydrating and uplifting mist.
- Reapply sunscreen and make-up.

Night
- Cleanse your skin to remove the dirt accumulated during the day. Use a light circular massage technique.
- Remove make-up, ideally with a muslin cloth soaked in warm water, then splash your face with tepid water.
- Tone, as in the morning.
- Use a night repair cream or face oil (see page 29). Again, apply in an upwards action.
- Have a drink of water and cool your bedroom before you nod off.
- On a weekly or fortnightly basis use a hydrating and deep-cleansing mask (see page 30).

Go natural

For a fresh, youthful glow, less is definitely more when it comes to skincare

How many products does it take to create your 'ready to meet the world' face? And of those, have you looked at the never-ending ingredients lists?

One of your skin's key roles is to provide a barrier, but that doesn't mean it's impenetrable. In fact, it's estimated on average we absorb almost 5lb of chemicals each year from the cosmetics and toiletries we use. Given that, on average, women use 12 products every day, containing as many as 175 different chemicals, it's no wonder your skin can start to feel and look 'overloaded'. It can't always cope with a constant bombardment by synthetic substances.

Of course, beauty companies aren't in the habit of making their skincare products deliberately toxic and, used in moderation, they won't have any detrimental effect. But if you're using 20 products a day on already sensitive skin, it can result in inflammation, irritation and accelerated ageing. Researchers at the University of Edinburgh have suggested that over-zealous bathing with harsh soaps and detergents may have contributed to a recent 40 per cent rise in cases of eczema in England.

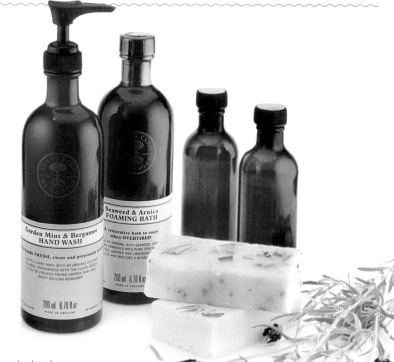

SIMPLIFY YOUR REGIME
The first step to going natural is to streamline your routine and avoid using two products when one will do. Give your bathroom cabinet an audit and get rid of any unnecessary – and money-wasting – extras.

DON'T OVERLOOK THE OBVIOUS
A skincare regime is important, but remember what you put *inside* your body is just as crucial, as is what your lifestyle's like. Before you slap on yet another product to deal with a complexion quibble, check your diet and daily habits aren't causing the problem. Dry skin? Ask yourself if you're drinking enough water. Lost your radiance and sparkle? Make sure you're getting adequate beauty sleep. You've only got yourself to blame if you're still smoking and have developed dark circles under your eyes. It makes sense all the things that energise

our bodies will also get our skin glowing, so address these.

CUT THE CHEMICALS

It's impractical to think you can avoid all synthetic chemicals. But you can give certain irritants a wide berth, particularly if you have sensitive skin. The bad guys include parabens, which are easily absorbed by the body and have been found to mimic the effects of female hormone oestrogen.

Sodium lauryl sulphate (SLS), a detergent that's added to shampoo, toothpaste and shower gel to boost lathering quality, can lead to severe allergic reactions. As can other petrochemical-derived ingredients including ethanol, also called ethyl alcohol, which is used to scent and colour, benzyl alcohol – used as a preservative – and acetone, which is an ingredient in some nail polish removers.

Another serious irritant is cocamide DEA (and cocamide MEA), a derivative of coconut oil, used as a thickener.

NATURAL WONDERS

Until recently, there's been a question mark over whether natural, plant-based creams are as effective as their high-tech counterparts. That's all changed. In the last few years, natural skincare companies, such as Neal's Yard and Dr Hauschka, have developed ways to combine scientific innovations in anti-ageing skincare with plant ingredients.

Research is proving how powerful these natural ingredients can be and even the cosmetics giants have caught onto women's desire for purity and are including more natural elements in their products. Look out for products that borrow from nature's store cupboard.

O Many valuable anti-ageing nutrients are also being used in beauty products. Antioxidant vitamins A, C and E, which help fight the free radicals involved in inflammation and ageing inside the body, can help battle acne, rosacea, wrinkles and pigmentation on the outside. Betacarotene – a member of the vitamin A family – has been shown to provide some protection against the sun. Even the most potent prescription skin preparation, retin A cream, used by doctors to fight fine lines and acne, is based on vitamin A.

O Plants and herbs have been used for centuries in nourishing skin recipes. Goji and açai, as well as rosehip and blueberry, are now the big trend in commercial skincare. They're all renowned for being rich in antioxidant vitamins. Meanwhile, soothing herbs, such as chamomile and calendula, can soothe inflamed skin.

O Natural plant oils, such as jojoba and argan, are much-lauded in skincare as they're far closer in composition to the skin's own oil (sebum) than synthetically made varieties. Essential oils lavender and frankincense are also deeply hydrating without the chemical load.

GO ORGANIC!

Organic products are not confined to your diet – you can give your skincare regime an organic makeover too. The Soil Association (SA) has developed rigorous standards system for health and beauty products, so you can guarantee the integrity of the products you use. Look for the trusted logos such as the SA's own, plus COSMOS ORGANIC and Ecocert, to ensure they meet strict organic standards. The SA's overriding principle is, if there's any doubt about an ingredient, it's banned – so their approved products are free of parabens, phthalates and GM ingredients. Look out for brands including Spiezia, The Organic Pharmacy, Green People, Weleda, Lavera, Inlight and Neal's Yard.

Natural and anti-ageing

When choosing natural skincare products, look for these naturally-derived anti-ageing ingredients.

O **Green tea** has a glowing reputation for helping to reduce the risk of cancer, and it could also boost your complexion due to its high levels of antioxidants called catechins.

O When used as a cosmetic extract, **pomegranate** has been shown to aid the regeneration of the skin's top layers.

O **Calendula** is packed with antioxidant carotenes and lutein, and is a renowned skin healer.

O **Chaga** and **pleurotis** mushrooms have potent anti-inflammatory properties, ideal for soothing skin.

O **Grape seed** is mildly astringent, so it can tighten and tone.

O **Pine bark** extract can help slow the breakdown of elastin and collagen and promotes good circulation.

O **Frankincense oil** can help balance your skin tone and is good for healing scars and blemishes.

O Used in after-sun products, **aloe vera extract** is anti-inflammatory and ultra-moisturising.

O Extracted from a Moroccan tree, **argan oil** is rich in vitamin E and essential fatty acids, and is great for hair and nails, as well as your skin.

O **Rosehip oil** is rich in vitamins A and E and essential fatty acids to boost hydration and suppleness.

O Used in ayurvedic medicine, **Gotu kola** is an anti-inflammatory herb said to slow collagen breakdown.

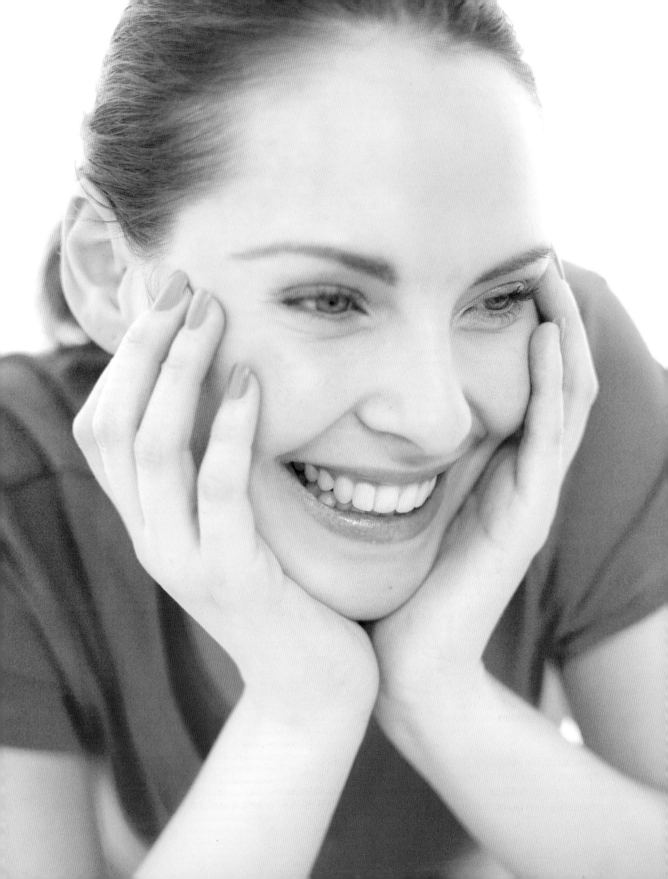

Anti-ageing skincare essentials

The star products you need to keep your skin youthful

The shelves of beauty departments are heaving with anti-ageing products, all making tempting claims. Before you splash out, here are the products that should form the foundation of your beauty regime, with top brands.

CREAM CLEANSER

Forget lather, think hydration. To leave your skin super-silky, choose plant-based products loaded with natural and nourishing extracts such as coconut oil, almond oil, hemp oil and shea butter. If your skin is oily, go for anything that contains non-astringent natural foaming agents and calming ingredients such as witch hazel and aloe vera.

TRY: Liz Earle Cleanse & Polish Hot Cloth Cleanser, Trilogy Very Gentle Cleansing Cream, Spiezia Facial Cleanser, Green People Gentle Cleanse, Elemis Pro-Radiance Cream Cleanser, Derma E Hyalauronic Acid Day Cream

ANTI-AGEING MOISTURISERS

This is the lynchpin in your regime to hold back the years. No cream will make you look 21 again, but a carefully-selected moisturiser can plump your skin, soften lines and increase radiance. Day creams should be loaded with antioxidant vitamins and plant oils, and unless you plan to get it elsewhere (for instance, from your foundation or primer), they should contain broad-spectrum UV protection.

TRY: Lavera Organic Restoring Day Cream, Neal's Yard Remedies Rejuvenating Frankincense Cream, Liz Earle Superskin Moisturiser, Origins VitaZing, Dr Haushka Regenerating Day Cream, Novostrata Regeneration Cream, Comvita Radiance Plus Moisturiser, Laura Mercier Flawless Skin

NIGHT CREAM

While you sleep, your body is furiously renewing itself – so it's the perfect time to indulge your skin with an intensive treatment. A night cream isn't always essential; if you feel your regular moisturiser does the job perfectly well, and so long as it doesn't contain SPF (obviously unnecessary at night), then don't feel under pressure to change your routine. However, if you regularly wake up with dry or taut skin, think about adding one into the mix. Try a luxuriant face oil (see page 30) or super-rich cream. Always thoroughly cleanse your skin before you apply it and don't forget to treat your neck and chest area too.

TRY: Weleda Wild Rose Night Cream, Trilogy Replenishing Night Cream, Vaishaly Anti-Ageing Night Cream, Oskia Bedtime Boost, Comvita Replenishing Night Moisturiser

EYE CREAM

The skin around your eyes is extra-delicate, so it deserves special attention. It's also where fine lines commonly first appear in your late 20s and early 30s. Peptides are common ingredients in anti-ageing creams, as are extracts of vitamins A, B5, C and E. Look for one with light-reflective particles if you're plagued by dark circles and SPF for day use. Eye creams are by their very nature lighter than regular moisturisers but opt for an even silkier gel product to tauten and douse morning-after-the-night-before puffiness. They're not always necessary but if your eye area is particularly dehydrated, try an extra-nourishing bespoke night-time cream. Always apply in a light, patting action with your ring finger to avoid stretching the skin.

TRY: Dermalogica Total Eye Care SPF 15, The Organic Pharmacy Lifting Eye Gel, Green People Eye Cream for Night, Dr Haushka Regenerating Eye Cream, Novostrata Regeneration Eye Cream →

FACE SERUMS AND OILS

Despite being packed with nourishing extracts, vitamins and essential fatty acids, these products are readily absorbed by the skin because of their small molecular structure. Serums are water-based and have lower oil content so are ideal for oilier skins and daytime use. Facial oils have a high concentration of essential oils and are perfect for night-time use when your skin can take an intensive hit. There's a product to suit every skin type; look out for products containing rosehip oil for mature skins and lavender for sensitive skins. Apply to clean, slightly damp skin, then massage in gently to stimulate circulation and aid absorption. After a few minutes, remove the excess with a cosmetic tissue.

TRY: **Jason Ester-C Hyper-C Serum, Estée Lauder Advanced Night Repair, Aromatherapy Associates Nourishing Face Oil, Aeterna Gold Collagen Crème Serum, Green People Rejuvenating Facial Oil**

HYDRATING MASKS

Treat your complexion to a regular mask. To protect your skin's hydration levels, steer clear of masks that dry out completely. If your skin is oily and needs a deep cleanse, kaolin clay and witch hazel are key ingredients. For a radiant pep-up, try products with extracts of brightening white or green tea and camphor. For the ultimate hydration, we recommend orange blossom, sweet almond and avocado oils.

TRY: **Nude Miracle Mask, Living Nature Hydrating Gel Mask, Aromatherapy Associates Overnight Repair Mask, Comvita Intensive Hydrating Mask**

GENTLE SCRUBS

Exfoliators, if selected carefully, can restore your healthy glow and give a feeling of 'newness' to your skin. Buffing particles of jojoba, rice enzymes and silica are gentle enough not to upset your delicate complexion. But if you have extra sensitive skin, try using a muslin cloth to wash away your cleanser.

TRY: **Liz Earle Gentle Face Exfoliator, Green People Brightening Exfoliator, Comvita Gentle Revitalising Exfoliant, Living Nature Vitalising Exfoliant**

LINE SMOOTHERS AND FILLERS

These are an (almost) natural alternative to cosmetic fillers. They temporarily 'blur' fine lines. Most feature microscopic particles of silicone and nylon, and come in pen-style applicators. Look out for lip plumpers that contain hyaluronic acid, peptides and capsicum, from chilli peppers.

TRY: **Nip + Fab Frown Fix, GoodSkin Labs Tri-Aktiline Instant Deep Wrinkle Filler, Trilogy Triple-Action Line Smoother, Eucerin Hyaluron-Filler Eye Treatment**

FIRMING BODY CREAMS

You'll never slim down with creams, lotions and oils alone, but firming and smoothing body products can smooth your legs, bum, stomach and breasts. Rich body butter is ideal if you're prone to dry skin. We recommend products loaded with gorgeous-smelling botanical extracts.

TRY: **Ren Wild Yam Firming, Smoothing Body Cream, This Works Really Rich Firming Lotion, Mádara Anti-Cellulite Cream**

BODY SCRUBS

It's impossible to shift cellulite completely but, in addition to toning exercise and regular body brushing (see page 47), invigorating scrubs can boost your skin's condition to improve its appearance. They're also great for rough, dry skin and for pre-tan prepping. Go for products based on natural oils, including olive, jojoba and almond, with stimulating extracts of essential oils, such as juniper, orange and rosemary.

TRY: **Origins Incredible Spreadable, Ila Spa Body Scrub for Energising and Detoxifying**

Super-scientific ingredients

Your guide to the latest high-tech skincare terms

○ **AHAs and BHAs**
Alpha hydroxy acids (AHAs) or fruit acids, such as citric and glycolic acids, and less harsh beta-hydroxy acids (BHAs), including salicylic acid, are exfoliating, brightening and can help iron out pigmentation and roughness.

○ **Retinol and retinyl palmitate**
As you'll discover in the diet section (pages 66 to 85), vitamin A is an important skin nutrient. These two ingredients (retinyl is better suited to sensitive skins) are topical versions of the vitamin, and enhance skin radiance and condition.

○ **Hyaluronic Acid (HA)**
A naturally occurring protein in your body's connective tissues that declines with age. When applied topically, HA can beef up your skin and fill out fine lines. It's popular in lip-plumping products.

○ **Peptides**
Combinations of amino acids and peptides are thought to promote collagen production and have firming properties.

○ **Ceramides**
These are lipids (fat and oil-like substances) that lock moisture into the skin.

○ **L-Ascorbic acid**
A stable, topical form of vitamin C that supports collagen production.

○ **Glycerine**
This draws and locks in moisture, to help hydrate dry skin.

○ **Alpha-lipoic acid**
A water and fat-soluble antioxidant that can give your skin a radiant glow.

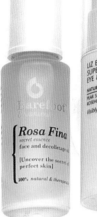
Barefoot
Rosa Fina
secret essence
face and decolletage...

[Uncover the secret of perfect skin]

100% natural & therapeutic

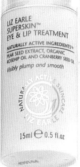
LIZ EARLE
SUPERSKIN™
EYE & LIP TREATMENT

NATURALLY ACTIVE INGREDIENTS
PEAR SEED EXTRACT, ORGANIC
ROSEHIP OIL AND CRANBERRY SEED OIL
Visibly plump and smooth

NATURALLY ACTIVE SKINCARE
LIZ EARLE

15ml e 0.5 fl.oz

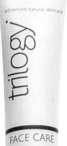
advanced natural skincare
trilogy

FACE CARE
eye contour cream

Restores and revives
the delicate eye area

certified organic rosehip
oil, aloe vera, vitamin A
and avocado

e 20ml
.67 fl.oz

laura mercier
flawless skin
REPAIR DAY CREAM SPF 15
CRÈME RÉPARATRICE DE JOUR FPS 15

LIVING NATURE New Zealand
harakeke and tree extract
firming
eye cream
to minimise the
look of fine lines
and wrinkles

10ml e 0.3 fl.oz

LIZ EARLE
SUPERSKIN
CONCENTRATE™

NATURALLY ACTIVE INGREDIENTS
ORGANIC ROSEHIP OIL, ARGAN
OIL, NEROLI OIL AND NATURAL
VITAMIN E

Visibly plump and smooth

NATURALLY ACTIVE SKINCARE
LIZ EARLE

28ml e 1 fl.oz

AGE PROOF
CoQ10 eye recovery
concentrate

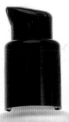

LIVING NATURE New Zealand
harakeke and rosehip oil
firming flax serum
to smooth and
soften fine lines

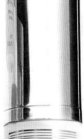
Skin
Science
Bio Active
Stimulating
Serum

e 30ml 1.06 fl oz

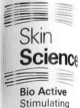

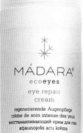
MÁDARA®
ecoeyes
eye repair
cream

regenerierende Augenpflege
crème de soin intense des yeux
восстанавливающий крем для глаз
atjaunojošs acu krēms

15ml/0.5 fl oz

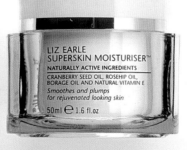
LIZ EARLE
SUPERSKIN MOISTURISER™
NATURALLY ACTIVE INGREDIENTS

CRANBERRY SEED OIL, ROSEHIP OIL,
BORAGE OIL AND NATURAL VITAMIN E

Smoothes and plumps
for rejuvenated looking skin

50ml e 1.6 fl.oz

Be beautiful for ever

Your skin has different needs in each decade.
Tailor your regime accordingly and you can look fabulous whatever your age!

Your skin changes markedly through the decades, from breakouts in your 20s and fine lines in your 30s, to loss of elasticity in your 40s, and sagging and dryness in your 50s and 60s. While a consistent skincare regime is essential throughout your life, subtle tweaks can help you manage these changes. Here's how to tailor your regime accordingly and look fabulous, whatever your age!

20s — Establish good skincare habits

Teenage discord gives way to plumpness and luminosity in your 20s, providing you have a healthy lifestyle.

Your skin's rate of cell renewal is on your side in your 20s, so this is the time to start a dedicated cleanse, tone and moisturise routine. Always remove your make-up before you go to bed. Ideally, avoid using cleansing wipes – they leave a residue of product on your skin. Use a gentle exfoliator regularly.

If your skin is still oily, use light moisturisers and oil-free make-up. Don't treat it harshly – abrasive products will strip out the natural oils and leave the upper layers of your skin dry and irritated. Your skin may still be prone to spots in your early 20s but if acne is a serious problem, see your GP and ask to be referred to a dermatologist. For skin scarred from acne, try massaging your skin with rosehip seed oil.

Don't drown your skin in products – invest in some quality key essentials that are based on natural ingredients. See page 26 for more advice on taking a natural approach.

Although your skin looks after itself, don't be complacent – damage it now and it will show later down the line. You may not see sun damage, but it could be accumulating on the sly, so use a daily moisturiser or foundation with a broad spectrum SPF protection.

Eat plenty of antioxidant-rich fruit and veg to keep your skin radiant. A homemade smoothie in the morning can help you reach your five-a-day – drink plenty of water to keep your skin hydrated, and minimise alcohol intake.

STAY YOUNG: Always use sun protection and follow a regular skincare regime to help prevent premature ageing.

30s — Adapt your regime as your skin changes

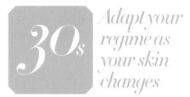

A decline in collagen and elastin, along with habitual expressions may cause fine lines to develop around your eyes, mouth and across your forehead in your 30s.

The delicate skin under your eyes thins and you may experience dark circles and puffiness. Add an anti-ageing eye cream to your regime and wear sunglasses to protect against the ageing effects of UV rays. Red spider veins may also start to appear – the cheeks are particularly vulnerable – so avoid using hot water on your skin and be religious about sun protection. If you have a hectic lifestyle, try to get lots of regenerative sleep and apply a vitamin-packed night cream.

Cell turnover declines and your skin will be duller than in your 20s, so use hydrating masks and gentle exfoliants regularly. Enlarged pores may be an issue so don't overload your complexion with heavy products.

STAY YOUNG: If your skin is looking dull, use hydrating masks and gentle exfoliants regularly.

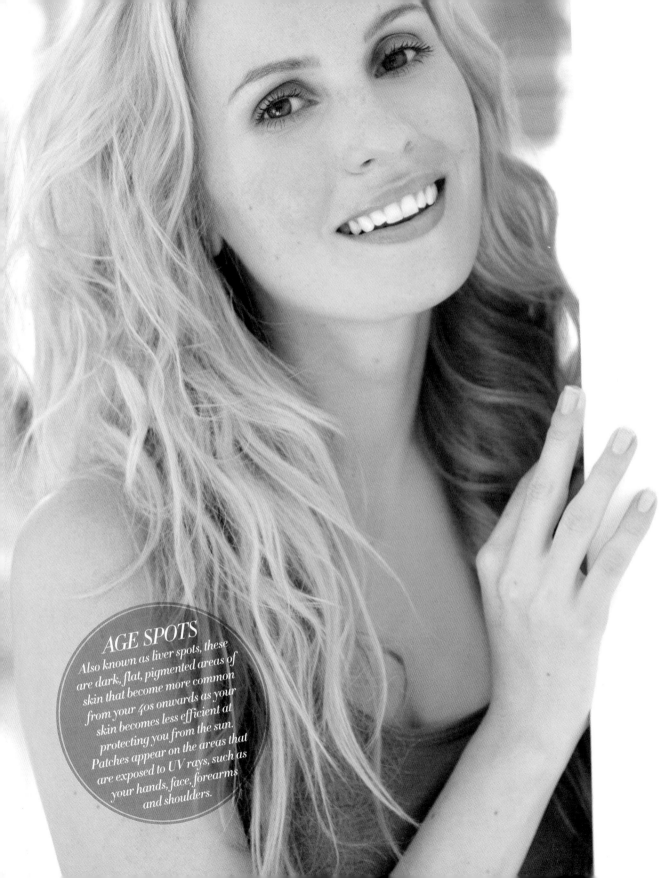

AGE SPOTS

Also known as liver spots, these are dark, flat, pigmented areas of skin that become more common from your 40s onwards as your skin becomes less efficient at protecting you from the sun. Patches appear on the areas that are exposed to UV rays, such as your hands, face, forearms and shoulders.

40s — *Protect against the onset of sagginess*

Cell renewal slows down when you enter your fifth decade, so give your complexion a helping hand. Try a face cream that contains alpha hydroxy acids (AHAs) and gently exfoliate on a regular basis. Your skin will appear much brighter and more youthful as a result.

Levels of your skin's natural oils (sebum) are likely to be lower now than in your 20s, so opt for creamy, hydrating products. If you had oily skin in your youth, you may find that it's more manageable now.

Because the skin's subcutaneous layer loses fat in this decade, your skin can lose some plumpness. Make sure you're getting enough essential fatty acids and phytoestrogens in your diet and look for anti-ageing products containing peptides and ceramides (see page 28).

Don't spend so much time on your face that you neglect your hands and neck – they are a classic age giveaway! Cleanse, exfoliate, tone and moisturise your neck regularly and use a moisturising handcream on your hands several times a day.

This is the age when you'll start to see signs of accumulated sun damage, such as age spots and crêpey skin, so always wear SPF cream (see page 45). Your skin will also be drier, particularly if you start to experience the first signs of the menopause, and blemishes will take longer to heal, so invest in regular facials.

STAY YOUNG: **Treat your complexion with respect, focusing on hydrating products such as luxuriant skin oils.**

50s plus — *Use ultra-rich anti-ageing products*

Your skin becomes thinner, less radiant and more translucent in your 50s, and, as oestrogen levels fall and oil glands contract, it may become more sensitive. You'll also be more prone to bruising. Avoid harsh treatments and allergens, such as perfumes, drink plenty of water every day and make sure you're getting plenty of healing and moisturising essential fatty acids in your diet.

If it's a jowly appearance that's the problem, try regular face exercises (see page 40) or lifting salon treatments (see page 46). Treat your skin with respect and upgrade your products across the board, including your make-up, to the most emollient (moisture-locking) types.

Age spots become noticeable now, so up your sun protection regime. You could try a salon treatment (see page 46) to help fade problem areas. Skin tags are common – about 50 to 60 per cent of over 50s experience them. If they're irritating you, see your GP, who can remove them fairly effortlessly.

To combat pigmentation and inflammation, avoid any foods (spices, alcohol and caffeine) that can cause flushing. Protect your skin in the elements, whether the weather is hot or cold. Switch to mineral-based make-up, redness-calming moisturisers and ask your doctor for advice if redness becomes a persistent issue.

STAY YOUNG: **Avoid harsh treatments and allergens, such as perfumes, and make sure you drink plenty of water every day.**

Care for your skin in pregnancy

Your skin changes in a number of ways during pregnancy and needs extra TLC.

First off, check your regular products are suitable. For instance, some (but not all) essential oils aren't safe to use. Ask your midwife for guidance if you're unsure. The hormonal tumult may make your skin extra sensitised or aggravate a long-standing skin condition such as eczema, so always choose gentle, extra-moisturising skincare products. You may find you develop more spider veins – a result of increased circulation and the softening of blood vessels, but rest assured they should largely abate post-pregnancy. An increase in skin pigmentation is also common during pregnancy, so take extra care to protect yourself with sunscreen. There's no clear evidence you can prevent stretch marks, but massaging your bump with a pregnancy-specific oil or lotion can, at the very least, make your skin more comfortable and it's relaxing too!

MAKE YOUR FAVOURITE SCENT LINGER LONGER

Just as you change your skincare products as you get older, change your perfume too. As skin gets drier, fragrances won't last as long as they once did. For extra staying power, choose pure perfume oils or, before you use your scent, apply a little moisturiser to the areas you want to spray to give the scent something to cling to. To find a new scent that's right for you, make sure you test it on your skin. Apply it to your pulse points and note how the scent develops.

Age gracefully

It's not just your face that needs TLC! Here's how to keep your whole body looking young

I t's every celeb's nightmare – you spend a fortune on your face and body only to be caught by the paparazzi showing wrinkly hands or a crêpey neck. Here's how to keep every part of your body looking the best it can.

HANDS AND NAILS

Cleaning, washing-up, gardening, typing… our hands have to cope with a lot. Because they're exposed to the elements and the skin's relatively thin, you may develop wrinkles on your hands in your mid-40s. As skin slackens and thins due to a drop in oestrogen and fat levels diminish, veins may become more prominent. Use hand cream – try an anti-ageing variety with SPF15. Get regular manicures with hand massages and wear gloves when washing up. Go for acetone-free nail polishes – always apply a base coat first, and massage your nails and cuticles regularly with natural oils such as jojoba.
TRY: Weleda Pomegranate Regenerating Hand Cream, Elemis Pro-Collagen Hand and Nail Cream, Barefoot Botanicals SOS Safety Gloves Barrier Hand Cream, Yes to Carrots Hand and Elbow Moisturising Cream.

BREASTS

Nearly 50 per cent of women in the UK are concerned about their boobs heading south as they age, according to a survey by bra manufacturer Triumph. Because breasts are mainly fatty tissue, you can't train them directly to resist the effects of gravity. However, you can tailor your fitness programme so you work your pecs and upper back muscles, which support the breasts and improve your posture. Always wear a bra when you're exercising, and make sure you're wearing the right-sized daily support too. Moisturise with a firming cream rich in antioxidants and essential fatty acids for an extra boost.
TRY: This Works Perfect Cleavage Firming Lotion, Palmer's Cocoa Butter Formula Bust Cream, Liz Earle Superskin Bust Treatment.

KNEES AND ELBOWS

The skin on your knees and elbows can get incredibly dry and pitted. Use a body scrub to slough off roughness and cosset in soothing, hyper-rich balms.
TRY: Ren Mayday Mayday Rescue Balm, The Body Shop Hemp Moisture High Balm.

FEET

Regular filing, scrubbing and deep moisturising are essential – there's nothing more ageing than a parched landscape of dry crevices on your heals. If your feet need some extra TLC, apply a deeply nourishing foot cream before bed, and sleep in a pair of cotton socks to maximise absorption. And don't forget sun protection when you're wearing open sandals. Regular pedicures are a must and always get issues such as corns professionally treated. Wear the right size of shoes and save stilettos and ballet flats for special occasions. They aren't supportive and can acerbate common issues such as hard skin, ingrown toenails, sensitive pads, blisters and back pain. Regularly stretch your toes and arches – massages, foot rollers and yoga classes can help.
TRY: Margaret Dabbs Intensive Treatment Foot Oil, Aveda Foot Relief, This Works Perfect Heals Rescue Balm.

GET A GLOW

An artificial tan can give you anti-ageing glow, provided it's applied well. Thorough prepping is vital. Exfoliate in the days before application, so your skin is buff and clear, and moisturise; this will help prevent your skin drinking up too much self-tanner. Give extra-dry parts such as elbows special treatment. Apply using gentle sweeping movements with flat hands – or use special tanning gloves – and don't forget hard-to-reach areas such as your back. If you aren't confident, use a dry mist rather than a lotion, or a gradual tanner to build up colour.
TRY: Lavera Sun Tan Lotion.

NECK AND DÉCOLLETAGE

In your mid-30s you may notice a loss of elasticity around your neck and upper-bust as your skin slows down its production of lipids. When you moisturise, include your neck and massage in an upward motion so you don't drag skin downwards.
TRY: Neal's Yard Rejuvinating Frankincense Firming Neck Cream.

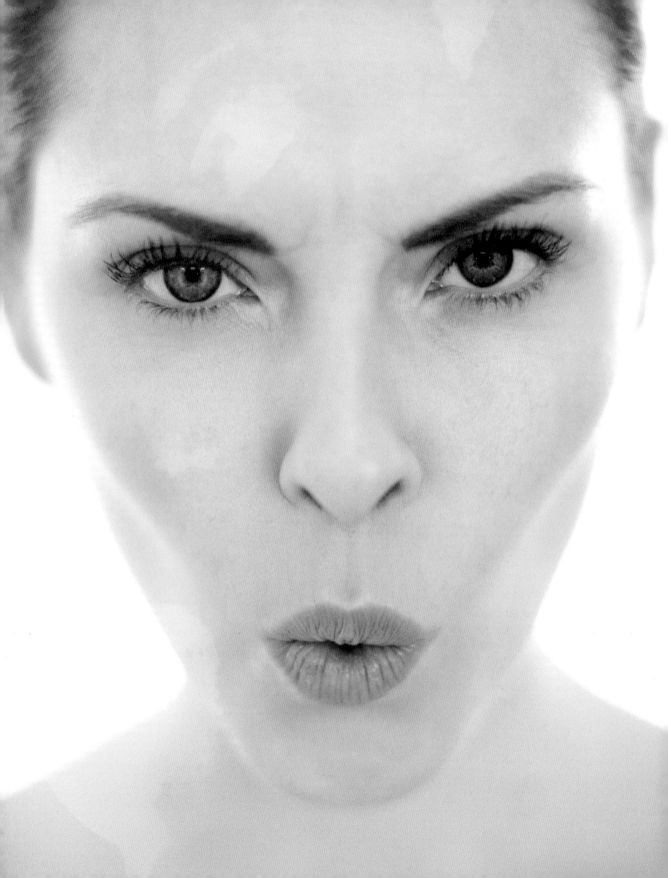

Keep your face fit!

Smooth away lines the natural way with a facial workout

We all know there's no cream in the world that will instantly give us a flat stomach, firm thighs or beautiful sculpted arms. The best way to get a fit body is through exercise. But when it comes to our faces, we happily rely on creams without regard for our facial muscles.

And yet, just as your body's muscles lose tone with age and underuse, so it is

> **A facial fitness routine can get your complexion in shape**

with the muscles in your face. Your facial muscles are directly attached to skin, so when muscle mass declines, unfortunately your complexion sags and hollows too. In the same way gym workouts keep your body toned, a facial fitness programme can get your complexion in shape.

FACE EXERCISE BENEFITS

Toning and strengthening the muscles under your face creates a natural lift. Facial exercise also improves circulation to the skin, bringing more oxygen and ➔

Work out with the facial exercise gurus

What personal trainers Matt Roberts and Tracy Anderson are to your body, these experts are to your face. Try out their methods using their books, workshops and one-to-one lessons.

○ **Eva Fraser** is the original natural facelift trainer, and developed the Eva Fraser Facial Fitness method in the 1950s. She believes just 10 to 15 minutes a day of facial exercise can help smooth out lines, firm up your jawline and 'lift' the face. Key exercises include 'face tapping' to boost circulation and under-chin slaps to lift the jawline. **www.evafraser.com**

○ Created by Finnish-born movement and dance specialist **Marja Putkisto**, the Method Putkisto Natural Face Clinic is based on the principles of yoga, Pilates and Alexander Technique. It's designed to work muscles you never knew you had, and alleviate the effects of poor posture. Her technique aims to unlock facial tightening by way of stretching and relaxation exercises,

which 'reteach' muscles, to reduce frowns and improve voice tone. The method is taught individually or in small workshops of up to 10 people. See **www.methodputkisto.com** for DVDs.

○ **Dr Hauschka Facial Gymnastics** combines 15 facial exercises with a natural skincare routine. A therapist examines your face and creates a customised programme for you. You then perform these exercises at least three times a week and apply the appropriate base cream for your skin type. **www.drhauschka.co.uk**

○ A hit with the likes of Gwyneth Paltrow and Madonna, Face Yoga combines established yoga postures with other facial exercises that not only benefit your face but boost your health in other ways. It's pioneered by New York yoga teacher **Annelise Hagen**. **www.yogaface.net**

○ Skincare expert **Marie-Véronique Nadeau** (www.mvorganics.com) is another exponent and author of *The Yoga Facelift* (Conari Press, £16.99).

nutrients – vital for a youthful healthy glow. And working your facial muscles improves lymph flow, reducing puffiness. Beauty experts believe the results you get from facial exercise are far preferable to cosmetic treatments. A filler, for instance, can treat a deep line but will still leave your skin slack. And regular injections of Botox, which freezes muscles, can cause them to start wasting.

So, what are you waiting for? Get a step ahead of the celebs and plump up your face the natural way. There's a whole range of techniques waiting to be tried – from face yoga to high-tech gadgets.

HOME TREATMENTS

If you fancy giving facial fitness a go at home, there are various gadgets you can invest in, should exercises sound like too much work! Popular brands include Slendertone Face (**www. slendertoneface.com**), Tua Trend facial wand (**www.tuatrendface. com**) and CACI face toning (**www. thefaceliftadvice.co.uk**), from the non-surgical facelift salon treatment experts. These devices use tiny – and safe – electric microcurrents to stimulate muscles, smooth out fine lines and restore plumpness and volume.

One study at the University of Galway found using Slendertone Face for 20 minutes five times a week for 12 weeks increased the zygomatic major (the smiling muscle) by an average 18.6 per cent. More than 90 per cent of women using the devices said their faces felt firmer and more toned. Researchers found the apples of the cheeks looked fuller and complexions became clearer and more radiant.

TRY THE FACE GYM

Alternatively, try an easy DIY face workout, to boost circulation to your complexion and douse the stress that causes frown lines in the first place.

Basic Stimulates all the facial muscles

○ With your back teeth lightly together, touch your face very lightly with your index fingers just above the corners of your mouth. Your lips should part slightly as you lift.

○ Smile using your cheek muscles, extending towards your temples.
○ Complete the smile incrementally, as if it's a six-step ladder, making sure you lift each muscle as your smile lifts.
○ Hold, then pulse your smile for a count of six. Return to the start in six movements also.

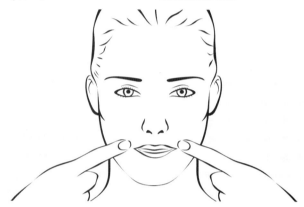

Eyelids Lifts your eyes

○ Place the pads of three fingers firmly across both of your raised eyebrows. Hold your hands slightly diagonally outwards.
○ Then, resting your fingers firmly on the browbone, blink six times.

○ Next, working against the resistance of your fingers, try to close your eyelids in four slow downward moves. Hold this exercise for a count of 10.
○ Relax for a few moments and repeat the exercise. But this time place the pads of your fingers on your eye socket bone without resting them on your eyelids.

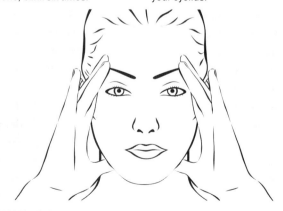

Forehead
Targets frownlines

○ Place your index fingers firmly along the length of your brows, which should be relaxed.

○ Then, moving against the resistance of your fingers, lift your forehead muscles without raising your eyebrows. Hold for a count of 10.

○ Finally, close your eyes and feel your forehead muscles slowly relaxing.

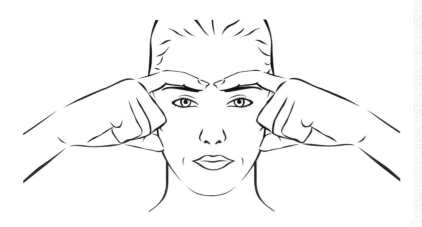

Ears Stimulates flow of blood to facial muscles and skin

○ With your index fingers and thumbs, hold the top rim of your ears and pull up. Using small rotations between your fingers and thumbs, massage the area.

○ Move down all round the rim of the ears to the lobe, pulling your ears out gently and massaging them.

○ Continue up to the top of your ear again. Repeat this for one minute.

○ With your index fingers, make brisk circular movements over the surface of the ears and massage all its crevices and spirals with the pads of your index fingers.

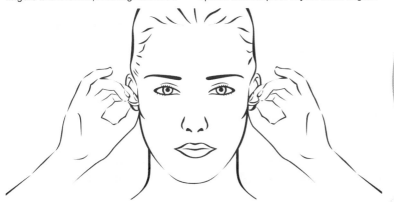

When we're het up, we crease our foreheads, squint our eyes and hold tension in our jaw, which pulls the corners of your mouth down. In addition to doing the following exercises every day after applying an intensive moisturiser, use light pinching all over your face to get the blood flowing and to feed your skin cells with nutrients.

Complete two sets of each of the Eva Fraser exercises on the left, once a day, for five days a week for best results.

BEAT COMPUTER FACE!

Too many hours in front of a computer screen can give you premature lines and wrinkles, warn beauty experts. Staring straight ahead at a 2D screen means our facial muscles aren't getting the natural workout they need. Our muscles naturally follow the movement of our eyes, so if you look upwards, your facial muscles and whole body responds and goes up too. Ensure you balance your time at the screen with plenty of activities, such as walking in nature and playing sports, which encourage healthy movement of your eyes and, in turn, your facial muscles.

A-LIST INSPIRATION

There are countless celebrities who've taken anti-ageing a bit too far. But there are plenty of fabulous role models who are handling ageing with aplomb. Looking younger than their years, but not unnaturally so are Julianne Moore, Gwen Stefani, Elle Macpherson, Michelle Yeoh, Susan Sarandon, Halle Berry, and Helen Mirren. We salute you!

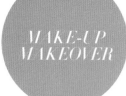
Make-up tricks

Want to look 10 years younger? It's easier than you think! The right products and techniques can take years off you

You wouldn't dare to wear the same clothes you did when you were a teen, and the same principle applies to your make-up. Just as your body shape alters and those hot pants may not be as appealing as they once were, so too the changes to your skin require a fresh approach to your make-up products.

Today's cosmetics can work wonders – from giving you dewy, fresh skin to concealing dark circles and blurring away lines. With a few choice products and clever make-up tricks, you can knock years off your face.

GIVE YOUR COSMETICS BAG A SPRING CLEAN

This is not simply to take years off your looks but to protect your wellbeing too! A recent survey by the College of Optometrists found 25 per cent of us use cosmetics that are more than four years old, putting us at risk of bacterial infections, including conjunctivitis. Experts recommend replacing mascara every six months and the main players – eyeshadow, lipstick and blusher – within two years.

GET A GLOW!

Dry, dull skin can make you look older. To recapture your youthful radiance, use a light-reflecting foundation – avoid flat matte – or a tinted moisturiser. Use a slightly damp brush to apply it and set with a fine and iridescent loose (not pressed) powder. Dab highlighter on your cheekbones, forehead and nose, and blend.

EVEN YOUR SKIN TONE

Sun damage and hormonal changes can upset the evenness of your skin tone. Thankfully, there's an array of corrector and primer products to use after moisturising and before layering on a light foundation. If you're suffering ruddy pigmentation, avoid red tones in your make-up, which will only draw attention to your problem.

BRIGHTEN YOUR EYES

Our eyes become smaller as we age. To brighten them, apply a light-reflecting concealer in the hollows under your eyes. Use a highlighter under your brows to add lift. If your eyelids are drooping, avoid blending deep shades into the sockets. Instead, start with a primer then apply a neutral shade to lighten and even your skin tone. Finish with eyeliner and mascara for definition.

MAKE LINES DISAPPEAR

Try one of the new magic line-smoother products. These generally include silicones and optical pigments that sit on the skin's surface and help blur the edges of your lines and wrinkles. Some products also include anti-ageing ingredients.

PLUMP UP YOUR CHEEKS

As we age, the youthful apples of our cheeks tend to slide downwards. Give your face an instant lift by applying a hint of blush onto your cheeks – the spot that plumps up when you smile. Opt for a cream blusher in a rose shade to recreate your natural, youthful rosiness.

The eyebrow facelift!

Tweezing your brows into shape is one of the easiest ways to add definition to your face. If you're not confident about plucking, get them done professionally – it's easy to keep the shape once you've been shown how. Invest in a good pair of slanted tweezers and pluck in decent light.

Hold a pencil vertically next to your nose – and remove any hairs that fall inside the pencil line. To work out where your eyebrows end, move the pencil at a 45° angle from your nose tip, so it's diagonally across your face. Remove anything below the pencil. Now work on the shape of your brow, by following its natural arch. Alternate which brow you pluck to get an even look. Thin brows are ageing, so make sure you don't overpluck.

PUCKER UP!

Like every part of your body, your lips lose tone over time. Add shape with a lip plumper containing hyaluronic acid. Outline with a neutral lip liner to add definition and prevent colour bleed. Shy away from matte lip colours, which can age you. Instead, opt for a light-reflective gloss to create the illusion of fullness. When you're in the sun, always apply an SPF lip balm.

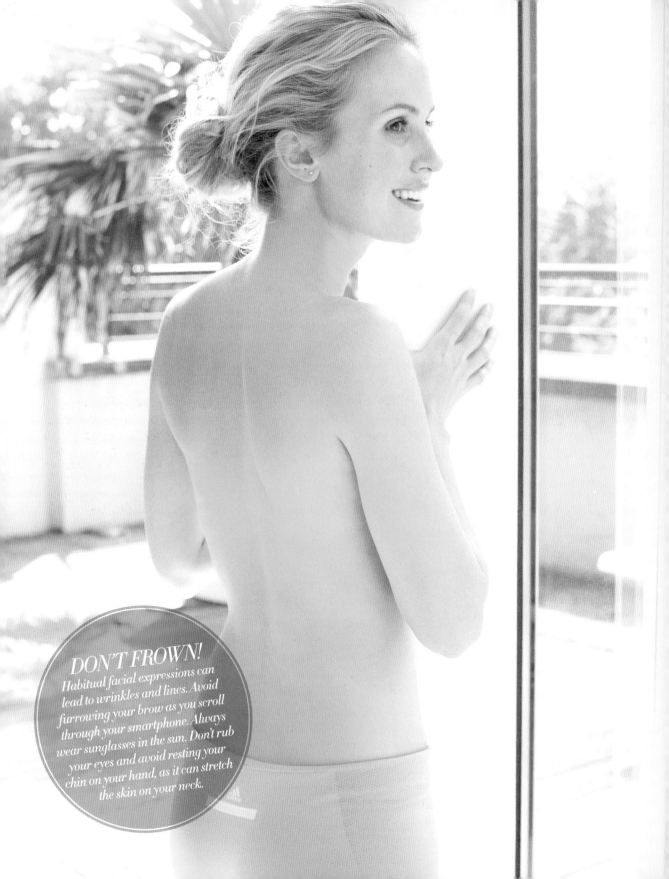

DON'T FROWN!
Habitual facial expressions can lead to wrinkles and lines. Avoid furrowing your brow as you scroll through your smartphone. Always wear sunglasses in the sun. Don't rub your eyes and avoid resting your chin on your hand, as it can stretch the skin on your neck.

Here comes the sun!

We all feel better when the sun comes out, but as it's the leading cause of premature ageing, it's good to know how to protect yourself

There are few things more uplifting than sunlight on your face – and a daily dose of sunshine is good for you. So much so that in 2010 several health bodies including Cancer Research UK and the National Osteoporosis Society issued new guidance, recommending we enjoy 10 to 15 minutes in the sun, without sunscreen, daily in summer to safeguard our vitamin D levels.

However, there's a fine line between safe and unsafe exposure. Apart from not smoking, protecting your complexion from sun is the most important thing you can do to prevent premature ageing. While UVB rays cause burning by damaging your skin's DNA, it's the UVA rays that are the main ageing enemies. They penetrate your skin and damage the structural fibres, which leads to photoageing – wrinkles and sagging. And prolonged exposure can increase your risk of skin cancer, one of the most common in the UK. Experts say it takes just one episode of blistering sunburn before the age of 20 to double your chances of malignant melanoma in later life.

PREVENT AND PROTECT

After a series of high-profile campaigns, public awareness about sun damage is greater than ever, but we're still, as a nation, woefully lapse about healthy sun habits.

Sun protection isn't just for holidays abroad. Daily face protection is necessary – even in winter sun. Sunscreens are added to many skincare products, but don't burden your complexion with multiple shields, as they can irritate. Choose one product, such as a daily moisturiser or foundation, that provides broad spectrum SPF15 protection, so it provides a barrier against both UVA and UVB rays.
TRY: **Trilogy Vital Moisturising Cream SPF15 and Jurlique Purely Age-Defying Day Cream SPF15.**

> *Be sensible in the sun. Wear sunglasses, a wide-brimmed hat and protective clothing*

In the UK, UVA protection is rated with a star system, varying from zero to five stars, so look for products with at least four stars. For more information visit **www.sunsmart.org.uk**.

Use a common-sense approach – if you spend the majority of your time outdoors you'll need something stronger than an office worker would use. If you have sensitive skin, try products with natural mineral filters.
TRY: **Lavera, Liz Earle and Jason. Try Green People No Scent Sun Lotion SPF25 and Neal's Yard Remedies Lavender Sun Screen SPF22.**

CHOOSE A HIGH FACTOR

If you're on your hols or relaxing outdoors in the summer sun, apply a strong broad-spectrum sunscreen liberally to all exposed body parts. Cancer Research UK recommends at least SPF15 with four stars or more, but has a 'the higher the better' message.
TRY: **Jason Sport Natural Sunblock SPF45 and Clarins Sun Wrinkle Control Cream UVB/UVA 50.**

Apply generously and regularly. If you sweat a lot or enjoy water sports, apply protection more frequently. Don't forget to cover the forgotten or hard-to-reach parts, including your ears, lips and the backs of your legs. And check the expiry date on your sunscreen! Some creams will only last 12 months.

The sun's rays can be stronger at high altitudes, and the snow reflects them back at you, so cream up when skiing.

No sunscreen can provide 100 per cent protection, so be sensible about exposing yourself to the rays. Wear a wide-brimmed hat, sunglasses and protective clothing and avoid sitting out between 11am and 3pm. Take care even if you're driving or sitting in a conservatory – windows don't block UVA and UVB rays completely.

Sunbeds are not a safe alternative to sunbathing and a fake tan won't protect you from sun damage – you'll still need to use sunscreen. And monitor your moles. Changes in size, shape or colour, bleeding and itching could be early signs of skin cancer.

Call in the pros

Your guide to the latest anti-ageing salon treatments

Sometimes professional expertise is called for. Maybe you have a special occasion coming up or a skin concern that isn't responding to your day-to-day beauty regime. Either way, calling on the skills of the experts can help you get the results you're looking for. Here's how to choose from what's on offer.

Facials

ELECTRO-STIMULATION
Tiny electrical currents are applied to your face to coax, tone and lift muscles, and enhance your skin's ability to neutralise bacteria and protect itself from daily damage. Used in conjunction with a relaxing facial.
TRY: **CACI (Computer Aided Cosmetology Instrument); Guinot Hydradermie Lift Facial.**

ACUPUNCTURE
Acupuncture points in your face are stimulated with tiny needles to increase the flow of blood and energy to the skin.
TRY: **Energy Bodies' Beauty Acupuncture; Annee de Mamiel Facial Acupuncture.**

MASSAGE
A blend of light acupressure and deep muscle stimulation wakes the skin and relieves tension.
TRY: **Organic Pharmacy Facelift Massage; Emma Hardie Natural Lift and Sculpting Facial; Neal's Yard Facial Rejuvenation Massage.**

OXYGEN
High-pressurised jets deliver oxygen infused with botanical and nutrient extracts to restore your glow.
TRY: **Bliss Triple Oxygen Treatment; Rani Mirza Oxygen Facial.**

PEELS
These use AHAs, especially glycolic acid, to stimulate cell renewal. They're not suitable for sensitive skins.
TRY: **Karin Herzog Peel & Plump; MD Formulations Glycolic Peel.**

Try a warm wax treatment where your feet are cosseted in layers of soothing wax

RESURFACING
Also known as microdermabrasion, micro particles exfoliate and regenerate the skin. Again, it's not recommended for sensitive skin.
TRY: **Elemis Tri-Enzyme Resurfacing Facial; Crystal Clear Microdermabrasion.**

AROMATHERAPY
As stimulating for your olfactory senses as your skin, these facials use anti-ageing essential oils and pampering massage techniques to hydrate and deep cleanse.
TRY: **Aromatherapy Associates Renew Rose Anti-Age Facial; ESPA Aromatherapy Facial.**

And for everything else...

CELLULITE
Of all salon treatments, cellulite-blitzing solutions are the most abundant. Choose from aromatherapy-based massage, high-tech 'bells and whistles' therapies, and everything in between. The most popular include Endermologie, a deep tissue massage using rollers and suction; manual lymphatic drainage, a rhythmic massage to pique the lymphatic vessels; and Ionithermie where a detoxifying thermal clay is applied to the skin and small electrical currents are used to stimulate the circulation.

UNWANTED HAIR
If you've tried all the other options (sugaring, threading, waxing, bleaching...) there are permanent solutions available. Electrolysis, where tiny electrical currents are directed into the hair follicles, is best for dealing with a small number of troublesome hairs, while laser treatment, which uses targeted laser beams to cauterise follicles, is available for wider areas, for instance underarm and lip hair. Several sessions are required.

THREAD VEINS
Microsclerotherapy is a popular non-surgical treatment for thread veins on the body and legs and is usually carried out by a medical professional. Over a course of 20- to 30-minute

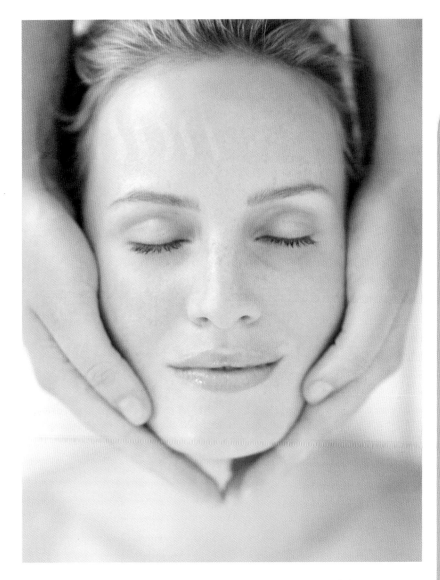

sessions, a fine needle is used to inject a 'sclerosant' solution into the veins. For troublesome facial thread veins, Intense Pulsed Light (IPL) laser treatments – also used for pigmentation and age spots – and electrolysis are recommended.

TIRED HANDS AND FEET

Your hands are constantly on show so deserve some expert attention too. Many of the specialist anti-ageing skin therapies we've mentioned above are available for your hands too – including IPL for age spots, electro-stimulation,

microdermabrasion and deep massage. For a general pep-up, try a hand treatment from one of the big beauty treatment players, including Elemis' Pro-Collagen Hand and Nail Treatment.

Acupuncture, oxygen therapy and massage can give weary feet a lift, but the star anti-ageing treatment is a medical-grade pedicure (medi-cure), normally carried out by a qualified podiatrist, to slough away hard skin. Alternatively, try a warm wax treatment, where your feet are cosseted in layers of soothing and smoothing wax.

Cellulite action plan

No one is immune to the dimply clutches of cellulite. Although a healthy lifestyle can improve its appearance, even svelte sporty types can have areas of orange peel skin. Commonly found on the hips, bum and thighs, cellulite is caused by fat deposits under the skin. Women are more prone to it than men as we have thinner skin and the connective tissue of our skin is slightly different. Gender aside, age, family history, hormones and lifestyle including smoking and diet can all contribute. Sadly, you'll never banish it entirely. However, regular attention can bolster your skin against tell-tale bulges. Treat your body to scrubs and ultra-hydrating creams, take regular exercise to rev up your circulation, manage your weight and eat a diet that's rich in fruit and vegetables, fibre, unsaturated fats and low in salt and processed foods.

Try daily body brushing:
O Before showering or bathing; use a brush with firm natural bristles to brush your body with long, smooth strokes towards your heart, starting with the soles of your feet.
O Pay attention to cellulite trouble spots – upper arms, bum and thighs.
O Don't forget your hands and armpits, shoulders and back.
O Follow with an energising scrub and slather on a rich body moisturiser or oil on your slightly damp skin. Look out for products with rosemary (not for sensitive skin), cypress and juniper oil, which are popular aromatherapy cellulite solutions.

Fabulous hair

Glossy, healthy hair is a sure way to make you feel amazing and get heads turning. Here's how to keep yours at its youthful best

We all know the difference a good – or bad – hair day can make to our mood and confidence. Healthy conditioned locks, plus a good cut and colour are key to keeping you looking young.

Your hair is very much a barometer of your inner health and wellbeing. If you're run down, dieting or stressed, it won't be long before it shows up in your hair. Likewise, the good news is that if you eat well, exercise, de-stress and get plenty of sleep, you'll soon see an improvement in your hair. Treat your hair well from the outside too. Overprocessing, whether with chemical treatments such as tinting and bleaching, heat treatments such as straighteners and tongs or overexposure to sun and chlorine can all take a toll.

Your hair is made from the protein keratin and is moisturised by your hair's oil, sebum, released from hair follicles in the scalp. Each hair is made up of overlapping layers of keratin. When the layers lie flat and smooth, your hair reflects the light, making it shine. When the layers are damaged, your hair is left looking dull and lifeless.

THINNING HAIR

Hair production gradually slows down as we age, so our hair naturally thins and dries. However, follicle foibles can strike at any age and, in total, it's estimated that 8 million British women are affected by some form of hair loss. Iron deficiency, pregnancy, some medications, autoimmune disease, episodes of stress or hormonal problems connected to the thyroid gland can trigger patches of baldness (alopecia) or overall shedding (telogen effluvium). Smoking can cause premature greying and thinning because it starves your follicles of youth-enhancing nutrients and oxygen. According to a study published

> **A good hair style can make you look 10 years younger and fill you with confidence**

in the *British Medical Journal* smokers are four times more likely to have grey hair and increased hair loss. Excess alcohol is dehydrating and can deplete levels of iron in your body. And stress can also trigger major hair loss. See your GP if you're concerned about the health of your hair.

ANATOMY OF GREY

If we were to ask you to name the key signs of ageing, we'd wager grey hair would be up there. Like your skin, your hair gets its natural colour from a pigment called melanin, and as we age the cells that produce it, called melanocytes, gradually slow. *Et voilà*, grey hair. Exactly when you go grey – and it's a gradual process – is very much determined by your genes. A recent Danish twin study published in the journal *PLoS ONE* showed that while hair-thinning on the top of the head in women is partly connected to environmental and lifestyle factors, greying is largely beyond our control.

That said, smoking and stress can accelerate it. Research done at Kanazawa University in Japan found that protracted levels of anxiety can damage the stem cells which help supply new melanocytes. While some may find their first grey hair in their 20s, greying usually starts in our 30s and 40s. No hair colour is out-and-out more prone to greyness but it shows up earlier on dark hair.

Keep your hair looking youthful

SOFTEN UP

A blunt, stiff or severe style can add years to your face, by drawing your eyes and cheeks down, so ask your hairstylist for some tousled layers to give your hair volume and your cheekbones definition. Have the best cut you can afford – a good hair style can make you look 10 years younger and fill you with confidence. Whether a maturing woman can carry off long hair is a great source

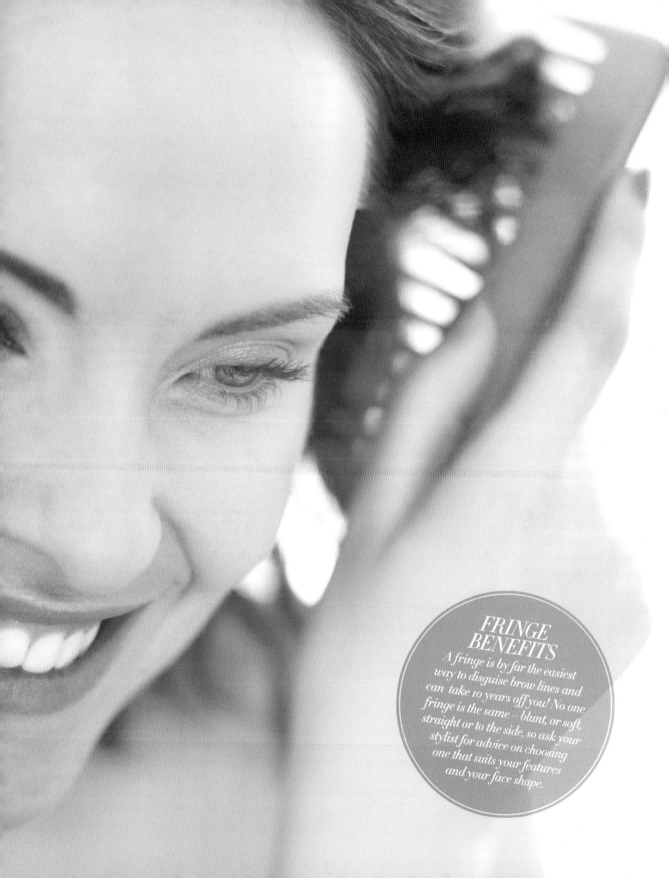

FRINGE BENEFITS

A fringe is by far the easiest way to disguise brow lines and can take 10 years off you! No one fringe is the same – blunt, or soft, straight or to the side, so ask your stylist for advice on choosing one that suits your features and your face shape.

of contention, but to be honest, you can carry off whatever style you want provided you look after it. Irrespective of the length of your mane, keep updating it and take indulgently good care of it.

COLOUR SENSE

Remember all the guidelines we gave you about your make-up colours? They're relevant to your hair too. Cover up grey, yes, but avoid harsh dye jobs, matt and unnatural shades. Go for soft colours that flatter your complexion – that means shades that are only a couple of shades from lighter or darker than your natural hair colour. Ideally, have your hair professionally coloured at a salon at least once to get advice on the best shade for your skintone.

There are some ultra-sophisticated techniques on the market – modern colourants are multi-toned and contain illuminating pigments that can transform ageing hair. If you're into natural products, check out Daniel Field's range of peroxide or ammonia-free dyes. Maximise your colour with colour-extending products, which contain UV protectors and are designed to seal the hair cuticle.
TRY: **Bumble and Bumble's range of bespoke products for blondes, redheads and brunettes.**

ADD VOLUME

Get your hair tended to regularly, the longer and more unkempt it is, the less bounce and swing it will have. For added oomph and depth, ask your stylist for a layered style. Try using big Velcro or heated rollers and techniques such as backcombing. And add some volumising products into your hair care regime.
TRY: **Phyto's Phytovolume range, the Thin to Thick range by Jason and Tresemmé's 24 Hour range.**

MOISTURE MUST-HAVES

As well as thinning, your hair gets drier over the years as oil production slows. Keep your hair glossy by avoiding straighteners and other scorching-hot appliances and dehydrating treatments, such as bleaching and perming. Protect your hair from chlorine by wearing a cap when you swim. Use replenishing intensive treatments and shine sprays regularly to bring back shine and make your hair more manageable. Natural-based products may help, as they don't contain moisture-stripping detergents.
TRY: **Mop's Glisten High Shine Pomade and the Dull/Lifeless Hair Kit from Green People.**

FEED YOUR HAIR

A chronic deficiency of iron, B vitamins and zinc can acerbate hair loss, so make sure you're eating a wide and balanced diet. Your hair is made from protein, so this is the most important food group for it. Essential fatty acids, present in nuts, seeds (or their oils) and oily fish, will help boost its condition. Add seaweeds such as arame, nori and wakame to your diet – use them in soups and stir fries – as they're rich in hair-friendly nutrients such as iodine, folate and magnesium. Consider a hair supplement if you need an extra boost.
TRY: **Vitabiotics Tricologic for Women which contains 26 nutrients including biomarine collagen, L-Cystine, iodine, copper and selenium.**

UV PROTECTION

Your hair and scalp are as susceptible to sun damage as the rest of your body. Over-exposing your hair to the sun can damage the molecular structure, so it can become brittle, dry and dull. For protection, wear a hat or scarf and apply UV-barrier sprays when you're out in sun.
TRY: **Schwarzkopf Bonacure Sun Protect UV Protection Spray.**

GO WITH THE FLOW

Good circulation to the scalp ensures your hair gets the oxygen and nutrients it needs to flourish. Regular aerobic exercise gives your circulation a kick-start and reduces stress, so is a must for healthy hair. A regular home scalp massage is a good idea. Using oil (see below), move your fingers over your scalp and neck in a small, but firm circular movements. Leave the oil in for 30 minutes, then shampoo and condition.
TRY: **For a home massage use John Masters Deep Scalp Follicle Treatment and Volumizer or a DIY mix of jojoba oil and a few drops of rosemary oil, slightly warmed.**

SOOTHE SENSITIVITY

Just as the skin on your body becomes drier and therefore more sensitive as you age, so does your scalp. Avoid chemical-laden products, heat treatments and abrasive dyes to help alleviate mild itching and flaking and try soothing scalp lotions or dandruff relief shampoos.
TRY: **Schwarzkopf Professional BC Bonacure Sensitive Soothe Scalp Serum or Jason Dandruff Relief Shampoo.**

SUPPLEMENT YOUR ANTI-AGEING DIET with some anti-ageing herbs. Amla (Indian Gooseberry) is an ayurvedic herb rich in vitamin C and anti-oxidants. As a tincture, take 30 drops up to three times a day. Milk Thistle can help support healthy liver function and the elimination of toxins – try it in tablet or tincture form. Gingko biloba has long been used to treat circulatory disorders and boost memory. Ginseng is revered for its rejuvenating and stimulating effects and research shows it can help prevent free-radical damage, but avoid it if you suffer from high blood pressure. Dong Quai Root (angelica) helps maintain healthy hormone balance and is a popular supplement during the menopause.

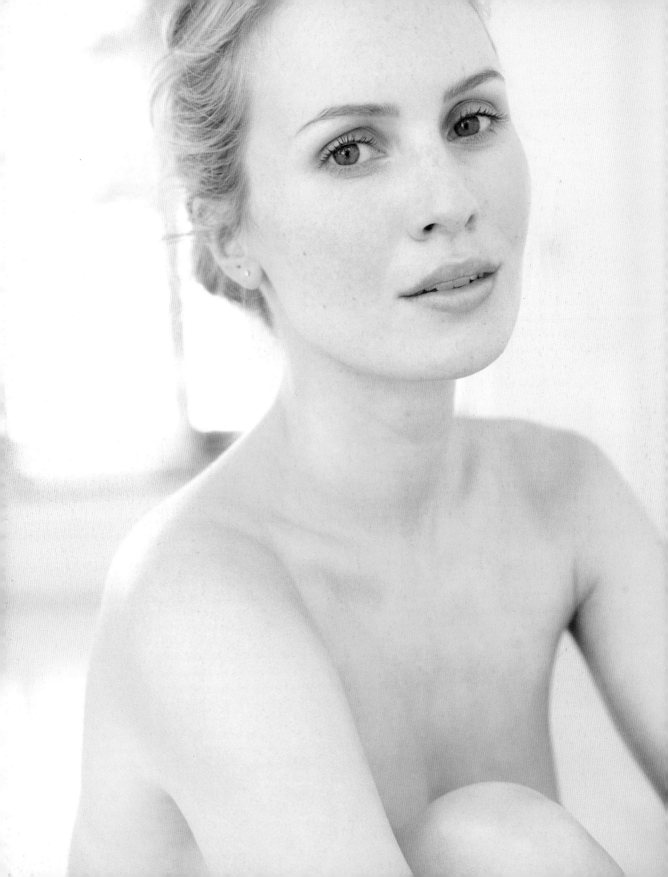

Your body

Your complexion is just the visible aspect of ageing. Passing years affect every part of your body in often unseen ways. This chapter is devoted to taking care of every nook and cranny – and the payback is you'll feel as young on the inside as you look on the outside. Find out how to look after your teeth, eyes and your joints. And take simple steps to protect your fertility, digestion and grey matter.

Beyond the wrinkles

Staying young goes further than just changing your skincare routine. Here's how to slow the signs of ageing that you don't see

We all worry about sagging flesh and body shape changes, but these are only the superficial signs of ageing. Hidden are some serious ageing factors that can affect your long-term health and wellbeing. But just because you can't see them, it doesn't mean you can't do anything to delay these changes. Here's what to do to stay young on the inside!

FERTILITY

Female fertility peaks in your early 20s. According to the Human Fertilisation and Embryology Authority, at 35 you're half as fertile as when you were at 25. Fertility drops dramatically after this – for women aged 35, about 95 per cent who have regular unprotected sex will get pregnant after three years of trying. At 38, only 75 per cent will do so.

Optimise your fertility with a healthy lifestyle. Being over or underweight can impair it – a certain level of body fat is needed to regulate the hormones that control ovulation and menstruation, so eat well and exercise. Eat foods rich in folic acid (green leaves), iron (red meat), calcium (dairy), zinc (seafood and asparagus), fibre (brown rice) and unsaturated fat (olive oil). Quit smoking as it can affect egg formation, ovulation and fertilisation, and don't drink excess alcohol. Stress can impact your reproductive system, so try yoga and meditation.

HEART

A strong heart goes a long way to helping you feel young. It is essentially a muscle, so it will lose strength over time, and as the blood vessels that supply it become less supple, it becomes less efficient. And your risk of heart disease

> **❝ Keep your heart young with a low-salt and low-saturated fats diet ❞**

rises after the menopause as levels of heart-protective oestrogen fall. If you have a family history of heart problems or stroke, be extra aware – the British Heart Foundation recommends you speak to your doctor about your risk from the age of 40 onward. Keep your heart young by following a diet low in salt and saturated fats, and don't smoke or drink excessively, or be a couch potato.

DIGESTION AND KIDNEYS

A well-functioning digestive system is key to everything from healthy skin to good energy levels. It slows down over time, but you can keep it young. Drink plenty of water every day and eat lots of soluble fibre. Research shows regular exercise aids digestion and can cut the risk of bowel polyps, which can lead to cancer, by up to 35 per cent. Chew food well and avoid huge meals.

Your urinary system also slows down, as the kidneys reduce in size and weight. You're more at risk of urinary incontinence with ageing, but keeping your weight in check and doing pelvic floor exercises can help.

LIVER

Your liver is a chemical processing unit, electricity plant and security guard all rolled into one. The liver performs more than 500 functions, such as breaking down food to make energy, combating infections and neutralising toxins. It's your largest internal organ and the most resilient – provided you treat it well.

Take care of yours by lowering your intake of alcohol and saturated fats. Excess drinking over a long period can cause cirrhosis, while obesity and a bad diet are linked to non-alcoholic fatty liver disease.

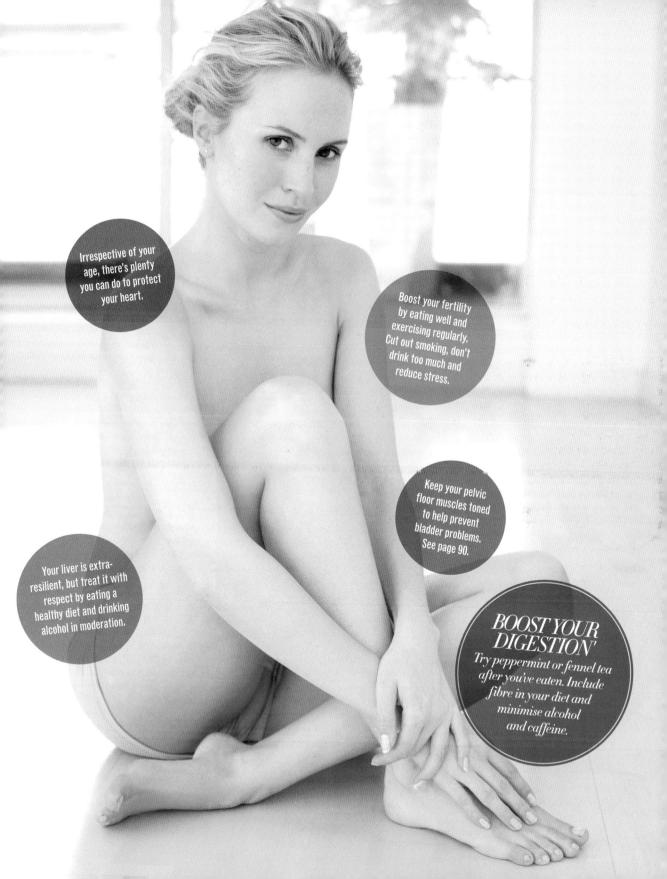

Irrespective of your age, there's plenty you can do to protect your heart.

Boost your fertility by eating well and exercising regularly. Cut out smoking, don't drink too much and reduce stress.

Keep your pelvic floor muscles toned to help prevent bladder problems. See page 90.

Your liver is extra-resilient, but treat it with respect by eating a healthy diet and drinking alcohol in moderation.

BOOST YOUR DIGESTION

Try peppermint or fennel tea after you've eaten. Include fibre in your diet and minimise alcohol and caffeine.

A youthful smile

There's nothing more ageing than yellowing teeth and receding gums, so time-proof your teeth now – and stay looking younger for longer!

G iven what we ask of them, our teeth are super-tough, but the natural ageing process takes its toll. And when it does, it can affect how youthful you look. When your gums recede and teeth darken and wear down, it can change the structure of your face, making you look older than you are. Gum problems can lead to tooth loss, and even cardiovascular problems, too, so looking after your oral health can pay off.

STAINED REPUTATION
As you age, the enamel on your teeth becomes more translucent and dentine – the layer beneath enamel – naturally darkens. Add daily consumption of staining foodstuffs into the mix and discolouration starts to appear. A dazzling-white Hollywood shine can look totally unnatural, but if you want to lighten the load on your teeth, try whitening toothpastes and speak to your dentist about professional treatments. It's best to avoid DIY home-whitening kits – research shows they can weaken your enamel. Instead, limit your intake of teeth-staining food and drinks (tea, coffee and red wine are the worst culprits), chew sugar-free gum after meals and always clean your teeth thoroughly.

BYE GUM
The risk of gum problems rises as you age, as accumulated bacteria grow in pockets at the root of your teeth, which can lead to infection and tooth loss. Practise good oral hygiene – floss and brush your teeth night and morning to remove plaque. Also, visit a hygienist twice a year for a 'deep clean'. Don't over-brush – gums naturally recede with age and this can accelerate it. Visit your dentist if receding gums have left any metal crown root pins exposed.

THE DAILY GRIND
Many people unwittingly 'brux' or grind their teeth at night. It can be hereditary or triggered by stress and can leave you with worn, extra-sensitive teeth. Your dentist should identify if you're a teeth-grinder and fit you with a night guard to prevent gnashing. Damage can be repaired with enamel veneers, but they're expensive and can be painful to have fitted.

DRY AND ARID
Hydration levels in your mouth plummet as you age. Because saliva works to neutralise acids, a dry mouth increases your risk of decay and gum problems. Chewing sugar-free gum after meals can help the problem and your dentist can recommend saliva-like mouthwashes.

Top teeth tips
Keeping your teeth youthful is all about common-sense habits.

○ Clean and floss your teeth twice a day. Have check-ups and professional teeth cleaning every six months.

○ When you're pregnant, your teeth and gums are more prone to problems – so good habits are important. You're allowed free NHS dental check-ups and treatment during pregnancy.

○ Minimise acid erosion. Keep sugary foods, fizzy drinks, acidic fruits and juices to a minimum.

○ After eating, sip on plain water and chew sugar-free gum to restore your mouth's natural pH level.

○ Temper your alcohol intake. Not only can some drinks damage enamel but excess drinking can increase your risk of developing mouth cancer.

○ Calcium is vital for strong teeth and omega 3 (in oily fish) is said to help dampen gum disease inflammation.

○ If you think you have an allergy from amalgam or silver fillings, which may show as ulcerated patches on the skin or mouth, see your dentist or GP.

GET A DENTAL LIFT

Inventors of a 'facelift brace' called Oralift (www.oralift.com) claim the device can reduce lines and jowls and firm the jaw. It does this by re-training the muscles in your face and jaw and boosting the flow of blood and oxygen.

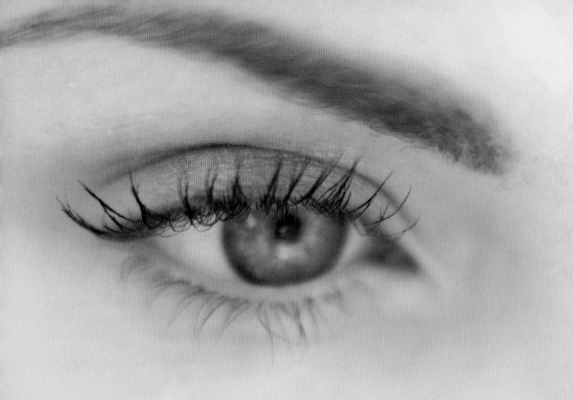

SCREEN SAVERS

If you're a regular computer user, give your eyes frequent breaks and remember the 20-20-20 rule: every 20 minutes, look 20 feet (six metres) away for 20 seconds to give your eye muscles a rest and help you blink more. And try some exercises to boost the supply of oxygen and nutrients to your eyes. Imagine a figure of eight, turned on its side, about three metres in front of you. Trace the figure with your eyes, without moving your head, in one direction, then the other. Next, hold your thumb six inches away from your eyes in front of your nose. Gaze at your thumb, take a deep breath, breathe out and focus on an object three metres away, then take another deep breath. Repeat frequently.

Vision on

Taking care of your eyes can help preserve your sight.
Here's how to keep age-related eye problems at bay

Diminishing eyesight is one of the most frustrating signs of ageing. After the age of 40, our eye muscles weaken and lenses lose flexibility, so it becomes harder to focus, see smaller objects or read tiny print. However, acute age-related eye problems can be reduced with a healthy lifestyle and regular check-ups. You need an eye test every two years, or more frequently if you wear contact lenses regularly, have diabetes or a family history of eye disease.

PARCHED PEEPERS

Your eyes become increasingly dry with age. Air conditioning, contact lenses, cigarette smoke, the menopause and a decline in optical hydration all play a part. This can trigger itching and even blurred vision and light sensitivity. Moisturising eye drops can help or ask your optician about 'artificial tear' drops.

Make sure you blink lots while you're working on a computer and consider buying a humidifier to moisten the air at home. Or try a more drastic treatment – tiny silicone plugs can be temporarily or permanently inserted in the tear ducts to reduce the speed at which tears drain.

BRIGHTEN YOUR EYES

Your eyes also start to look duller, puffier, and bloodshot as you age. Brightening up your eyes can make you look years younger with very little effort or sacrifice. Get plenty of quality sleep, moderate your alcohol intake and avoid cigarette smoke. For an instant lid-lift, apply cucumber slices or cotton wool pads soaked in rosewater and refrigerated.

AVOID SUN DAMAGE

Prolonged exposure to sunlight can damage your eyes, especially the retina and lens. Research shows it's linked to an increased long-term risk of cataracts – cloudiness in the lens – and may

> **❝ Brightening up your eyes can make you look years younger with little effort ❞**

trigger age-related macular degeneration (AMD), the leading cause of blindness in the UK. Always protect your eyes on sunny days, particularly if you're by the sea or pool or on a snow-capped mountain – both water and snow reflect glare and can increase the UV rays entering your eyes.

Quality sunglasses will also protect the skin around your eyes and prevent eye-scrunching, which can aggravate crow's feet. Look for glasses that offer UVA and UVB protection, with a CE mark or British Standard BSEN 1836:1997, which mean they conform to current recommendations. Protect your eyes with safety goggles during DIY and with sports glasses for activities such as squash.

COSMETIC TRICKS

Make-up can also help enhance the youthful appearance of your eyes, or make you look older if you're not careful. Avoid dark, heavily frosted or glittery eye shadow as you age – it can make the whites of the eyes look duller. Think softer, lighter colours with a mild shimmer. As the eyelid skin sags, your eyes can appear smaller. Counteract this by using softer make-up, abstaining from eyeliner on your lower lids and employing a pair of lash curlers to open up the eyes. Get those tweezers out – maintain your natural brow arch to give your eyes a lift.

FEAST YOUR EYES

A startling 65 per cent of us could be at risk of future eyesight problems because we're unaware that what we eat affects it, according to research from the College of Optometrists. Studies show that a balanced diet, rich in antioxidant vitamins A, C and E, lutein (a nutrient) and omega oils may help protect against eye diseases, including AMD. So tuck into leafy greens, peppers, oranges, blueberries and sweetcorn. Watch your weight too – obesity is linked to eye problems.

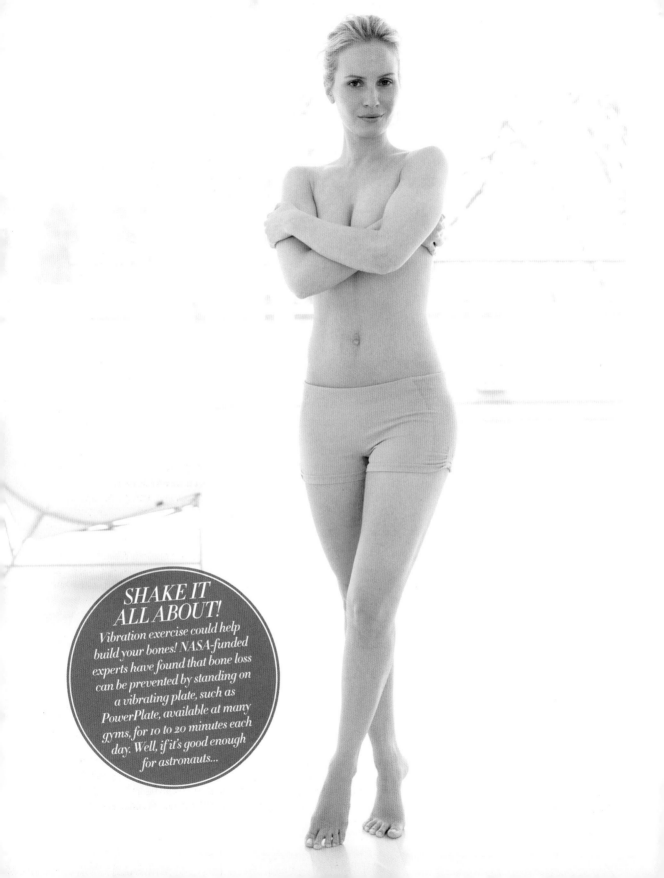

SHAKE IT ALL ABOUT!

Vibration exercise could help build your bones! NASA-funded experts have found that bone loss can be prevented by standing on a vibrating plate, such as PowerPlate, available at many gyms, for 10 to 20 minutes each day. Well, if it's good enough for astronauts...

Joint effort

Staying flexible and strong will help you look and feel younger,
so start taking care of your bones and joints now

You may think your bones stop growing after your teens but they're constantly being renewed, albeit more slowly, in adulthood. Your skeleton renews itself every seven to 10 years, though it took just two when you were a child.

BOOST YOUR BONES

Bone strength is usually inherited from your parents and it declines after the menopause – one in two women over the age of 50 will break a bone, mainly as a result of osteoporosis. However, more controllable factors can contribute – a sedentary lifestyle and excessive exercise, smoking and low levels of vitamin D and calcium compromise bone density. Even though you build your peak bone mass in your early 30s, it's never too late to strengthen them.

A study published in *Medicine & Science in Sports & Exercise* found that, even in postmenopausal women, strength training not only prevents the loss of density, it also builds bone matter in your spine and hips. Here are the best ways to boost your bones:

○ **Stay a healthy weight.** Being both under or over your optimum weight can put your bones at risk.

○ **Exercise regularly.** Do weight-bearing exercise, such as jogging, dancing, tennis and power-walking, for at least 30 minutes a day. Exercise will also help you manage stress – high levels of the stress hormone cortisol can damage your bones.
○ **Eat a calcium-rich diet.** Aim for 700mg a day, equivalent to a 200ml glass of milk. Leafy greens, tinned fish, fortified cereals and soya foods are other good sources.
○ **Eliminate your vices.** Stick to the daily alcohol limit of two to three units, swap caffeine for herbal teas and drink plenty of water – up to eight glasses a day.
○ **Get your vitamin D fix.** You need this vitamin to absorb calcium and the best source is sunlight. Aim to get 15 minutes of sun on your skin every day in summer, so your body can store enough for winter.

KEEP YOUR JOINTS YOUNG

We tend to only notice our joints when something goes wrong, but looking after them now will keep you flexible and youthful in the years ahead. Joints become stiff and creaky over time – knees and hips are particular trouble-spots because they carry lots of weight.

Age-related inflexibility is down to two major factors – our ability to produce joint-lubricating synovial fluid declines, and cushioning cartilage becomes stiffer and less flexible, so bones may begin to

rub together. Minerals may also deposit in and around some joints in a process called calcification. Here's how to keep your joints young and healthy:

○ **Stay a healthy weight.** The more pounds your joints have to carry, the more strain they're under. According to experts, almost 20 per cent of people aged 25 to 34 have a 'joint age' of over 50 because they're carrying excess weight.
○ **Prioritise exercise.** Focus on tennis or yoga where you shift your body in multiple directions. This will mean your joints will be able to cope better with falls and uneven ground. Weight-training also helps strengthen the supportive muscles and ligaments surrounding your joints, so the pressure is taken off them.
○ **Change your diet.** Studies show that omega 3 fatty acids in fish oils and pumpkin and sunflower seeds can help reduce the inflammation that may contribute to joint pain. Also, eat leafy greens – scientists at the University of East Anglia have discovered a compound found in broccoli and cabbage, called sulforaphane, blocks the enzymes that cause wear and tear on the joints. Although more research is needed to assess its benefits, many people find that glucosamine and chondroitin supplements help ease joint pain.

Mind games

Follow our brain-boosting tips and keep your little grey cells on tip-top form

Having a lively, active mind is one of the keys to staying youthful. And the good news is that everything from what you eat to who you talk to can help improve your brain function. Age-related brain drain starts so gradually, you may not even notice it happening. As the number of brain cells (neurons) decreases, even from a fairly early age, nerve impulses sending messages across the brain slow down and our ability to do simple things, such as remembering names and multitasking, wanes. According to research at the University of Virginia, in the US, reasoning, spatial visualisation and speed of thought decline in our late 20s and memory dwindles from our late 30s onwards.

But, it's not all doom, gloom and mental confusion. Research shows that keeping fit, healthy and mentally active can slow decline and even stimulate positive changes. In fact, science now shows that we can grow new neurons and neural pathways and regenerate the brain. The cognitive abilities you derive from accumulated knowledge increase up to the ripe old age of 60.

STAY ACTIVE
Regular exercise protects your brain from ageing as it helps to control blood pressure and weight, both of which influence cognitive functioning as you age. However, it has far more sophisticated benefits too. A Swedish study published in the journal *The Lancet Neurology* found that exercising for half an hour at least twice a week during midlife can reduce the risk of dementia by about 50 per cent. Scientists believe that by boosting circulation, exercise can flush the brain with nourishing blood and oxygen and

> **❝ Experts found having close friends and family protects against dementia ❞**

help keep its complex tissues healthy.

Your exercise programme doesn't have to be adventurous, simple yoga inversions increase blood flow to the brain, and, according to a study led by University of Pittsburgh, in the US, simply walking six to nine miles a week can help preserve brain size.

USE IT OR LOSE IT
Tasks that stimulate your brain can help maintain memory and cognitive processing. A study of cognitively healthy older adults in the *Journal of the American Geriatrics Society* found those who trained their brain were able to improve their auditory information

processing speed by about 58 per cent (versus seven per cent in controls). And you don't need to buy expensive 'brain training' gadgets to keep your mind in eminent condition. A report by *Which?* suggests crosswords, learning a language, memorising poetry or playing standard computer games may be as just as effective.

STAY SOCIABLE
Proving that good health isn't all about effort and sacrifice, an active social life has been shown to age-proof your brain too. Experts at the Rush University Medical Center in Chicago, in the US, found that having close friends and staying in contact with family members offers protection against dementia. In fact, the study showed that many people with Alzheimer's who had good social networks didn't suffer from the clinical manifestations of the illness, such as cognitive impairment or dementia. If friends and family don't live nearby, join a local group so you feel more part of your community. A running group or regular yoga class will have the added fitness benefits, as well as linking you with like-minded people.

FEED YOUR MIND
While you can't reverse the brain drain with diet alone, experts agree that eating well is phenomenally effective

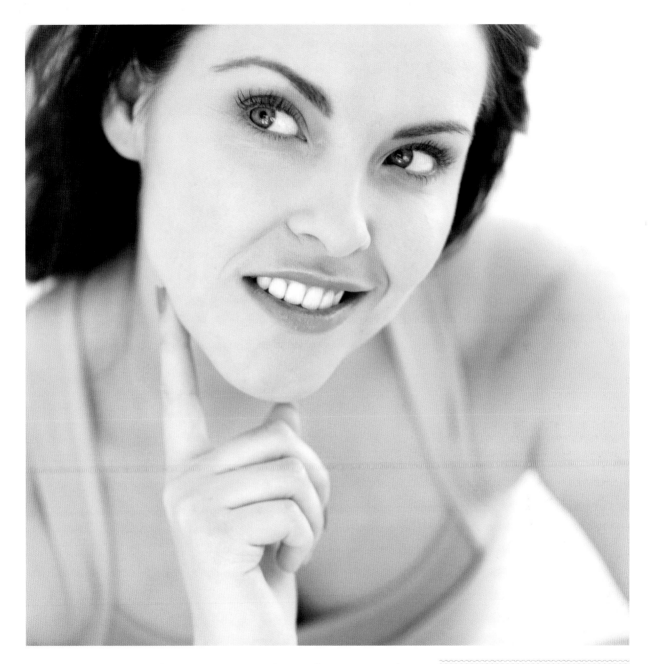

for keeping your grey matter firing on all cylinders. The B vitamins, found in wholegrains and nuts among other foods, are vital – research at Oxford University recently showed they can halve the rate of brain shrinkage associated with dementia. The much-lauded omega 3 oils found in oily fish are also essential – they're high in DHA, a fatty acid thought to support the nervous system. And, not forgetting antioxidants, lycopene (found in tomatoes) and vitamin E (present in nuts, seeds, cereals and eggs) are celebrated for their ability to mop up free radicals. Your brain is a hungry beast, so on a day-to-day basis, don't skip meals or rely on stimulants such as sugar and caffeine. Eat a diet rich in low-GI slow-energy release carbs, such as brown rice to keep it stoked up.

GO GREEN

Drinking green tea could protect your brain against dementia, finds a study by Newcastle University. Green tea contains health-boosting compounds called polyphenols, but scientists didn't know if they survived the digestion process. But the study confirms that they survive and also bind to proteins known to play a role in the development of dementia, hence protecting the brain.

Perfect posture

Want to look instantly slimmer and younger? Just make some simple changes to the way you carry yourself

One sure way to add years to your appearance is to hunch your shoulders and stand badly. We're naturally more susceptible to twinges in our shoulders, neck and back as we get older. And long-term

Walk with your head up, shoulders back, tummy in and a shorter stride

poor postural habits, such as slouching and hunching, along with a sedentary lifestyle all combine to make you look older than you really are. But treating your posture with a little TLC won't just ensure you stay enviably mobile and flexible – there is a multitude of additional benefits. It can help you look slimmer and improve your breathing, so you look and feel calmer and more confident. In essence, good posture enables your body to function better. Deskbound jobs, heavy handbags, driving, laptops and sky-high heels – many aspects of

HEAD AND NECK
Create length between your ears and shoulders by lengthening the top of your head towards the sky at all times.

SHOULDER GIRDLE
For good shoulder posture, imagine you're sliding your shoulder blades down towards the back of your waist, opening your chest naturally.

YOUR CORE
Your transversus abdominis muscles are your own built-in corset – to engage them, gently draw your navel to your spine.

NEUTRAL SPINE
Your lower back should be neither arched nor flattened, but somewhere in between. Maintain your back's natural curves.

LOWER BODY
With your weight in the centre of your feet, draw yourself up, as if creating space between the joints of your ankles, knees, pelvis and spine.

modern life – are damaging our posture. Here are some tips on how to behave more courteously towards yours…

WHAT'S YOUR TYPE?

First, discover your posture type by standing sideways on to a mirror to check the position of your pelvis and shoulders. Seventy per cent of us stand in a sway-back posture with the pelvis tipped back, a result of spending too much time sitting down. However it's positioned at the moment, you need to bring it back underneath you, in order to keep your spine in alignment.

For those with a sway back, squeeze your bum and tuck under your tailbone (at the base of your spine), making sure your lower back still retains a gentle curve. Gently pull in your tummy, focusing on the area between your belly button and pubic bone, and check your beltline is horizontal or near to it. Bring your shoulder blades back, then broaden them out down your back as much as you can. Pull your chin in slightly, as though it were being pulled in from the back by a ventriloquist – your earlobes should be above your collarbone.

STAY SWITCHED ON

Maintain sound posture at all times. From the car to work to the sofa, many of us spend the best part of the day sitting down. It's important to take regular breaks from your recumbent position, but also practise the right way to align your body when you *are* sitting to prevent back and neck problems.

Ensure you head is stacked vertically above your sitting bones – jutting it forwards can stress your neck and upper back. Make sure your earlobes stay in alignment with your shoulders. Roll your shoulders back and down. Keep your feet flat on the floor (avoid crossing your legs), shoulder-distance apart and knees level with or just below your hips – use a specially designed foot-rest if you need to. Both your hips and knees should be bent at 90°. Try to keep your body soft and don't sit up too stiffly.

WALK TALL

When you walk, hold your head up, bring your shoulders back and pull your tummy muscles slightly in. You're aiming to walk lightly, so shorten and soften your stride. Your head should be tall and not looking down – dropping your head puts a lot of tension on your neck. To see where you're going, drop your eyes without dropping your head.

If you have to carry a bag, make it as light as possible and use alternate sides, or even better, use a backpack so your arms are free. High heels cause your pelvis to tip forward and your head to jut out to compensate for the misalignment. Don't wear them for protracted periods and always choose supportive footwear for walking.

POSTURE FIT

Staying active – in any way – is brilliant for your posture as it strengthens the muscles that work to support your spine and pelvis. However you choose to keep fit, maintain a relaxed, open posture and activate your core by imagining you're trying to stop yourself weeing.

For targeted postural benefits, try a holistic mind-body technique. Pilates and yoga are great for working your core – the corset of supportive muscles around your midriff. Meanwhile, Alexander Technique can re-teach you how to sit, stand and walk in an effortless and co-ordinated way. And, according to researchers from Bristol and Southampton universities, it is a *bone fide* way to manage back pain.

Body shapers

Try these instant fashion tips to disguise your trouble spots.

○ **Hips and thighs:** Go for wide-leg trousers in dark colours. Avoid clingy dresses and boxy, short jackets and tops. Opt for ruffles or bold patterns and jewellery on your top half. Try full-skirted dresses.

○ **Upper arms:** Ditch sleeveless tops – and capped and fitted short sleeves. Three-quarter length and long fluted sleeves are a godsend. Wear a statement bracelet or cuff to emphasise narrow wrists.

○ **Stomach:** Shun skinny trousers and pencil skirts. Interesting necklines and chunky necklaces draw the eye upwards. Try low-waisted jeans and flat-fronted trousers or flared skirts to elongate your shape.

○ **Bottom:** Choose wider-legged or flared trousers and jeans but avoid back pockets. Structured, tailored dresses can sculpt. Draw attention away from your behind with detailing on the front. Wear long-line tops in non-clingy fabrics – go for A-line skirts and coats. Avoided pleated skirts.

○ **Legs:** Sharp tailoring on your bottom half is more flattering than loose styles. Again, draw the eye upwards by top-half colour or detail. Avoid shoes with ankle straps. Try maxi-length skirts or dresses – or shorter hemlines with long boots.

○ **Chest:** If you're well-endowed, opt for V-shaped or sweetheart necklines to lengthen your neck. Avoid smock tops and dresses and anything too tight. To draw attention to your bottom half, choose floaty skirts.

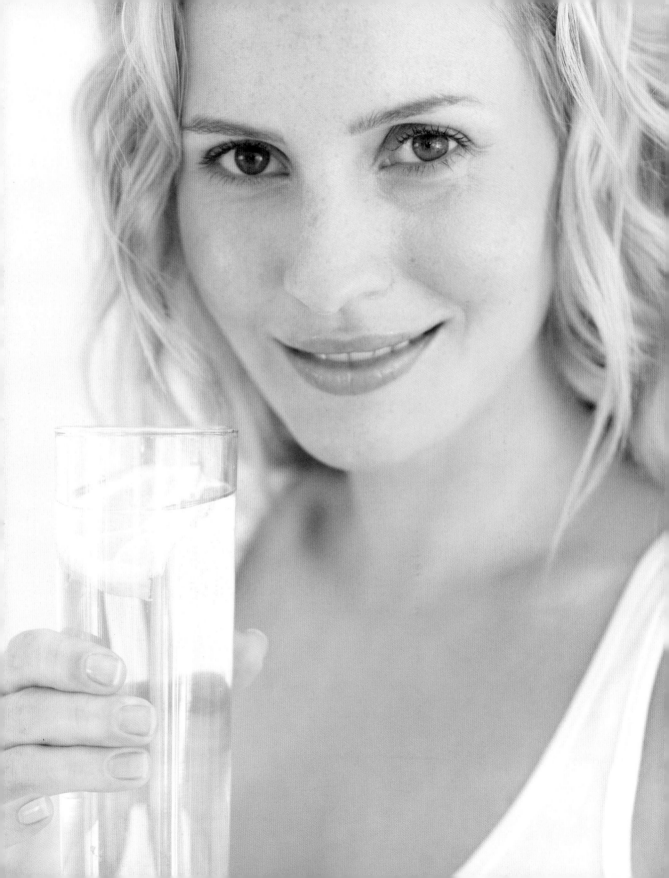

Your diet

The benefits of a healthy, wholesome diet filter to every part of your body. It can extend your life too – research published in the Journal of the American Dietetic Association shows people who have a diet of mostly vegetables, fruit, wholegrains, low-fat dairy products, fish and poultry live longer than those who indulge in junk food. In this chapter you'll find out about stay-young superfoods, how to feed your skin and eat for your age.

Feed your face

A nutritious diet doesn't just boost your health and reduce your risk of age-related disease, it can make you look more youthful too. Here's how to eat to boost your looks

We've all been through periods in our lives when we haven't had the time or inclination to eat healthily. And you don't need us to tell you that it shows on your skin almost immediately. It stands to reason – the skin is your body's largest organ, it's constantly renewing itself and it's nutrient-hungry.

Now scientists are discovering more about the complex relationship between complexion and diet. Many experts, including the world-renowned dermatologist Dr Nicholas Perricone, author of *The Wrinkle Cure*, believe the typical western diet is a major cause of wrinkles. In particular, Dr Perricone singles out our love of sugar and simple carbohydrates, such as white bread, as a problem area. He argues that a sugary diet encourages collagen fibres (which should keep your skin springy and firm) to stiffen in a process known as glycation, leading to visible ageing.

Your skin relies on a nourishing supply of oxygen from your blood. So, as well as avoiding sugar, anything that compromises your circulation – in particular saturated and trans fats – are a big no-no. As are dehydrating tipples, such as alcohol and caffeine.

Conversely, research is showing certain foods such as antioxidant-rich fruit and vegetables and omega-3-rich oily fish can boost skin by reducing inflammation (a key cause of ageing in our skin and body) and fighting free radicals.

RECIPE FOR SKIN SUCCESS

A skin-boosting diet should include all the food groups, (fats, carbs and protein) plenty of water and be replete in antioxidants to fight free-radical damage and boost your immune system.

> 66 *Fish oil can help reduce sun damage, thinning of the skin and wrinkles* 99

BOOST YOUR COLLAGEN

It's important to feed your body with the nutrients it needs to produce and maintain its scaffolding tissue – in other words, protein and vitamin C. Eggs are great anti-agers – as well as being a great source of protein, they also contain the detoxifying amino acid cystine, which aids the formation of collagen. Vitamin B1 (thiamine) has also been shown to slow down the loss of collagen fibres, so up your intake of vitamin B-rich wholegrains, including brown rice, and eat more oatmeal and sunflower seeds.

HYDRATE AND KEEP INFLAMMATION AT BAY

Two to three litres of water a day is a must – more if you're in hotter climes or exercising rigorously. In addition, essential fatty acids (EFAs) available in fish, nuts and seeds can help maintain your skin's hydration levels. There is some evidence that fish oil can help reduce sun damage, thinning of the skin and wrinkle formation. We know that EFAs have calming, anti-inflammatory qualities too, as do B vitamins, so stock up on wholemeal pasta, nuts and seeds, fish, chicken and avocados.

PROTECT YOUR CELLS

Antioxidants are foremost in your battle against ageing skin. A good antioxidant rule-of-thumb is to eat a rainbow of vividly coloured fresh fruit and vegetables. Dark green leafy veg, blood oranges, red grapes, carrots, squash and red peppers are all super potent. Pack in berries, cherries and green tea, which all contain proanthocyanidins, which are antioxidants, plus green veg for free-radical scavenging carotenoids, and tomatoes and red fruits for lycopene, which helps reduce inflammation and protects skin from UV damage.

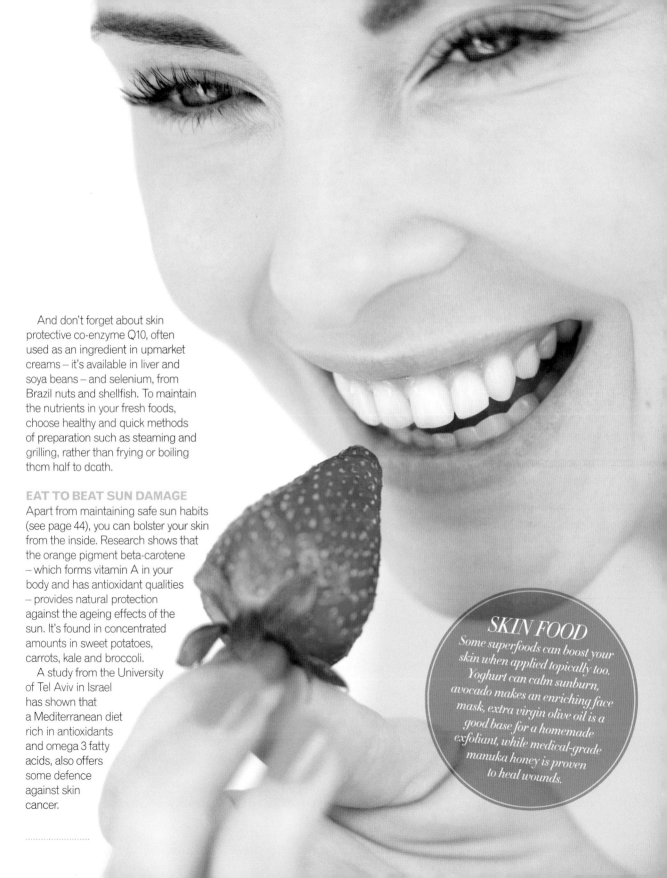

And don't forget about skin protective co-enzyme Q10, often used as an ingredient in upmarket creams – it's available in liver and soya beans – and selenium, from Brazil nuts and shellfish. To maintain the nutrients in your fresh foods, choose healthy and quick methods of preparation such as steaming and grilling, rather than frying or boiling them half to death.

EAT TO BEAT SUN DAMAGE

Apart from maintaining safe sun habits (see page 44), you can bolster your skin from the inside. Research shows that the orange pigment beta-carotene – which forms vitamin A in your body and has antioxidant qualities – provides natural protection against the ageing effects of the sun. It's found in concentrated amounts in sweet potatoes, carrots, kale and broccoli.

A study from the University of Tel Aviv in Israel has shown that a Mediterranean diet rich in antioxidants and omega 3 fatty acids, also offers some defence against skin cancer.

SKIN FOOD

Some superfoods can boost your skin when applied topically too. Yoghurt can calm sunburn, avocado makes an enriching face mask, extra virgin olive oil is a good base for a homemade exfoliant, while medical-grade manuka honey is proven to heal wounds.

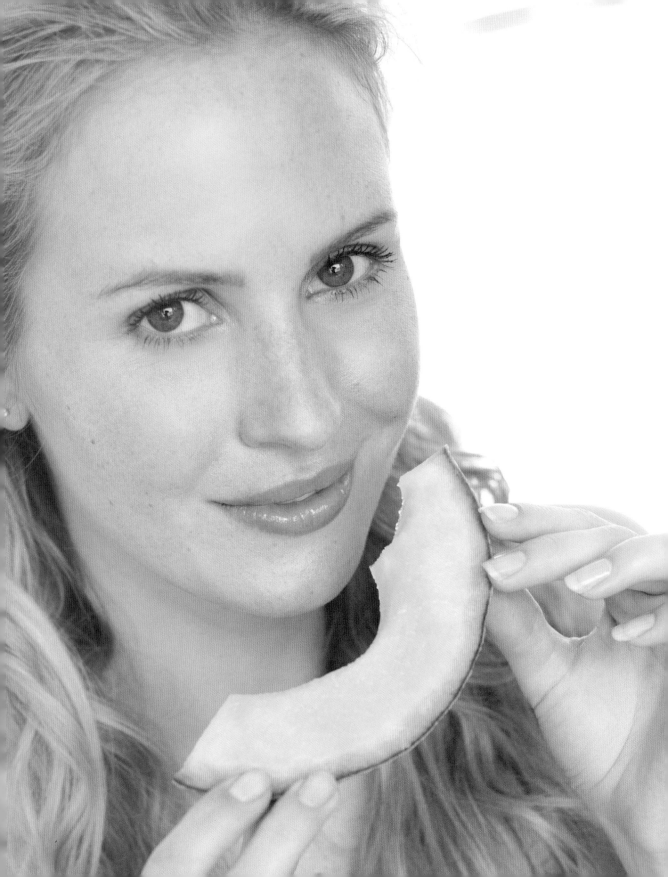

Stay-young superfoods

From blueberries to tomatoes, there's a wealth of wonder foods
that will help you look and feel full of vitality

Eating to hold back the years is all about having a balanced diet every day, so we're reluctant to highlight any individual foods. However, some are so potently anti ageing, they deserve their time in the limelight. Here's our pick of the best.

OILY FISH

Protein-rich and abundant in omega 3s, oily fish, such as salmon, mackerel, anchovies and sardines, can help to boost your skin tone, lubricate your joints, halt the brain drain and protect your vision. Researchers at Tufts University, Boston in the US believe that oily fish could offer protection against the eye disease, age-related macular degeneration, by altering fat levels in the blood after a meal that can be damaging to the body. Eat two to three times a week.

BERRIES

From açai to blackberry, bilberry to goji, berries are superlative anti-agers. They're brimming with antioxidants called anthocyanins, which benefit everything from your heart to your skin. A Chinese study published by the American Society for Nutrition has shown that berries can lower levels of bad cholesterol (LDL) and up the good one (HDL). Meanwhile, research presented to the American Chemical Society has found that the high levels of natural compounds called polyphenolics found in berries can activate your brain's natural 'housekeeper' mechanism, which cleans up and recycles toxins linked to age-related memory loss and other mental decline. Add liberally to your morning muesli or blend into a smoothie.

> 66 *Berries are full of antioxidants, which help everything from your heart to your skin* 99

ALLIUMS

Consisting of garlic, onions, leeks and chives, this humble family of plants is one of wrinkle guru Dr Nicholas Perricone's favourites because they're rich in anti-ageing antioxidant flavonoids. Garlic is top of the class – it's shown to have additional anti-viral, anti-bacterial and anti-fungal benefits and is thought to boost heart health and circulation, plus bolster your immune system.

FLAXSEED

Eaten whole, sprinkled on to salads and muesli or as oil, flaxseed is a great vegetarian source of essential fatty acids. Also known as linseeds, flaxseeds are rich in alpha linolenic acid (ALA), a type of omega 3 fatty acid. Studies show ALA is heart-protective, can help reduce joint inflammation and boost your brain.

GREEN TEA

We've mentioned it a couple of times already – but forgive us because the anti-ageing benefits of green tea know no bounds. It's been shown to possibly lower cholesterol, elevate brain function and protect against cancer. One study from the University of Alabama in the US has suggested that drinking green tea may actually help reverse the DNA damage caused by excess sun, linked with both wrinkles and skin cancer.

BEETROOT

It used to have a staid school-dinner image but beetroot is enjoying a

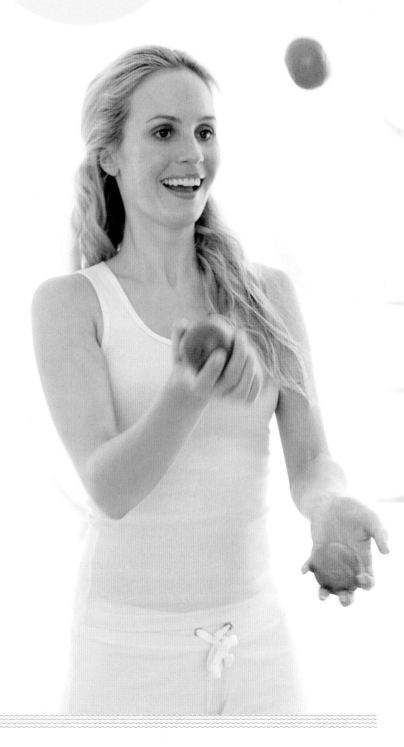

nutritional renaissance on account of its high levels of antioxidants and power nutrients, including sodium, magnesium, potassium and vitamin C, and betaine, which is linked to good heart health. A study from Wake Forest University, North Carolina in the US has found that the nitrates in beetroot can boost blood flow to the brain, keeping your mind sharp and potentially safeguarding against cerebral decline.

NUTS

A source of muscle-building protein, fibre, essential fatty acids and anti-inflammatory B vitamins, nuts pack a mighty nutritional punch. Study after study also shows that they can help in cholesterol management and therefore prevent heart disease.

But don't over-indulge, since they're high in calories, and eat them in their natural form rather than roasted or salted. Brazil nuts get a gold star – they're rich in selenium, which helps block the formation of an enzyme involved in ageing, which is produced in response to air pollution.

TOMATOES

As well as being vitamin C-rich, tomatoes contain a health-enhancing natural pigment called lycopene. It's been shown to defend your skin against UV damage, lower the risk of prostate cancer in men and offer heart protection.

PULSES

They're not as glam as blueberries and salmon, but the pulse family, including lentils, chickpeas and kidney beans, is

---

A LITTLE OF WHAT YOU FANCY DOES YOU GOOD!

Research published in *Chemistry Central Journal* confirms that chocolate is a rich source of antioxidants. Go for 70 per cent dark varieties for maximum impact. The odd glass of vino is no bad thing either – red wine contains a shot of heart-boosting anti-ageing goodies, including resveratrol.

rich in anti-ageing nutrients. They're low GI, so they drip-feed the body energy. They're also rich in fibre, potassium and zinc, plus they're a fab source of muscle-building protein. Add them to soup, stews and salads.

MANGO

The vibrant orange flesh of this exotic fruit is a supreme storehouse of vitamin C and most notably of beta-carotene, which is a key skin saviour. It's fibre-rich and also contains traces of minerals, including magnesium, calcium and phosphorus.

SOYA PRODUCTS

Soya milk and tofu are rich in oestrogen-like substances called isoflavones, which help maintain collagen and skin softness, and may help to balance falling levels of oestrogen as we become older. Like fish and pulses, they're also a great protein alternative to meat as they're free of saturated fats. Tofu is a valuable source of calcium.

GREENS

The chlorophyll that makes greens green is an anti-ageing wonder. Leafy vegetables are rich in vitamin C, calcium, iron, folate (vital for healthy blood vessels) and an eye-boosting nutrient called lutein. A study published online in the *British Medical Journal* recently found that eating greens regularly can significantly reduce the risk of developing type 2 diabetes.

But it's not just vegetables we should be quaffing. Green plant extracts, including wheat grass and algae varieties spirulina and chlorella, are super-rich in protein, as well as anti-ageing nutrients beta carotene, B vitamins, iron, potassium, zinc, magnesium and phosphorous.

Supplementary benefits

Nutritional supplements are in no way a substitute for a healthy lifestyle, so if you suspect your diet is remiss, address what you eat as a first line of action. However, if you do decide that you need an extra nutritional boost, remember that you need to take supplements daily and be patient about visible results. They should complement healthy habits, rather than replace them.

Studies show that our food may be less nutritious than it once was, so a catch-all A to Z multi-vitamin could be particularly helpful for redressing a shortfall of essential nutrients including minerals selenium, magnesium and zinc. Popular brands include Solgar and Centrum.

There are various bespoke skin, hair and nail supplements on the market – look out for brands including Perfectil, Viridian and Imedeen – which contain cocktail of complexion-boosting nutrients, commonly beta-carotene, grape seed extract, lycopene, evening primrose or starflower oils, vitamin E, vitamin C and zinc. These nutrients have benefits that extend beyond your complexion. For instance, lycopene has cardiac benefits and zinc is essential for the immune system. Because of the breadth of ingredients in them, you don't need to take a general multi-vitamin alongside a skin supplement.

A myriad of single nutrient supplements may try have knock-on benefits for your skin. These include co-enzyme Q10 (brands include Healthspan) – a naturally-occurring substance that's present in all bodily cells but declines with age; probiotics (BioCare) to aid your gut health and improve your body's ability to eliminate waste and absorb nutrients; supergreens and algae (try Sun Chlorella or Pure XP), rich in protein, antioxidants and essential minerals such as iron.

We've mentioned omega oils and they benefit not just your skin, but your heart and brain too. If you feel you don't pack enough into your diet, there are plenty of options on the market including Udo's Choice, Efamol and Nature's Best. Hyaluronic acid, a plumping ingredient used in skincare products (check out pages 28–31) is also available as a supplement (try Viridian, Solgar or Higher Nature). And collagen, the substance that acts as your skin's scaffolding is also available in capsule-form – try Proto-Col's range.

To balance your hormones, which can improve your skin, try widely-available evening primrose and starflower oil supplements, which are brimming with (GLA), an omega 6 essential fatty acid, and supplements of phytoestrogens, such as soy isoflavones, that work by mimicking oestrogen in the body and are therefore ideal to take in your 40s.

ANTI-AGEING ENEMIES

As well as avoiding sugars, salt and processed white foods, try to moderate salt and your intake of red meat – studies have linked excess to heart disease and cancers, including bowel and breast cancer. Watch your consumption of saturated animal-derived fats, such as butter, and hydrogenated or trans-fats, artificially created fats present in fast food, some margarines and mass-produced baked goods. Choose healthy methods of cooking such as grilling and steaming, and eat charred, barbecued foods in moderation as they contain carcinogenic compounds.

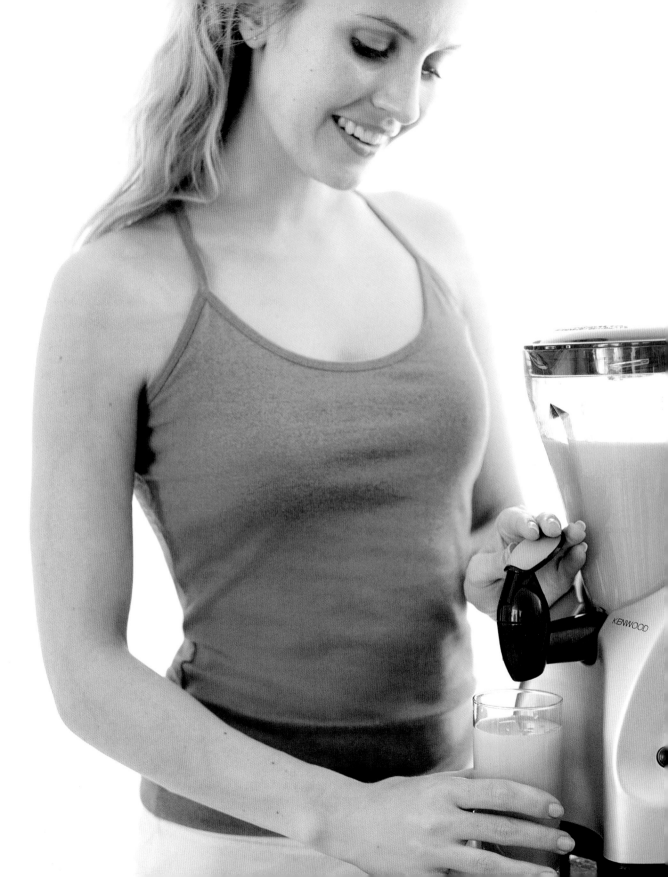

Eat for your age

Your decade-by-decade healthy eating guide for a slim and youthful body

An age-appropriate diet can help you stay feeling and looking your best, while laying down good health foundations to meet the challenges of the next decade. Here's how to eat your way to a healthy head start in the anti-ageing stakes.

This is the time to capitalise on your body's natural good health. Your bone density, muscle mass and metabolism peak in your 20s, so treat them with respect and build up a bank of reserves for the future. To feed your bones, eat a wide range of calcium-rich foods, including dairy and tinned fish. To bolster your muscles, pack in healthy protein, such as eggs, nuts, pulses, tofu and lean meat. Iron deficiency is common in young women – leafy greens, dried fruit and red meat should redress the imbalance or see your GP for advice. This is likely to be your party-hard decade so watch your alcohol intake – it's calorie-laden, dehydrating and can disturb your sleep. Try not to skip meals or overdo takeaways – fast food needn't be unhealthy if you sharpen your cooking skills. Balanced, regular meals will keep your mood and energy levels constant.

Prevent the natural decline of muscle mass (and slowing metabolism) by eating plenty of protein. Maximise your fertility (see page 54) by keeping alcohol to a minimum and eating folate-rich foods, including leafy greens and fortified wholegrains. Start looking after your heart. Swap saturated fats for plant oils, reduce your salt intake and up your fibre consumption. Watch your weight as it'll get harder to shed the pounds as you age. Stock up on healthy essentials such as brown rice, pasta, tinned tomatoes and pulses, nuts and seeds. Fine lines can show in this decade, so make sure your diet is brimming with antioxidants – available in green tea and brightly coloured fruit and veg.

The pounds can creep on in your 40s, especially around your belly. This happens as muscle mass and levels of oestrogen dip, which encourages weight to gather in your midriff. As well as resistance training (see page 90), a balanced diet will help counteract this. Watch your portion sizes – you need fewer calories with each decade as your metabolic rate slows. Maximise your metabolism with regular meals, and eat lean protein and low-GI carbohydrates, such as wholegrains. Along with fruit and veg, wholegrains will ensure you get enough fibre to protect your heart and your digestive system. Your risk of breast cancer increases, so minimise alcohol and, as the menopause approaches, get enough calcium and vitamin D to nourish your bones. Include phytoestrogens in your diet – available in soya products – as they can help recoup some of your body's natural decline in oestrogen.

Following a healthy diet from a young age pays dividends now – but it's never too late to change. What you eat now can delay age-related diseases, such as dementia, and could reduce your risk of certain cancers, including bowel and breast. After 55, you have a greater risk of atherosclerosis, where the blood vessels lose elasticity and start to clog, increasing your risk of stroke and heart attack. Continue to eat a cardio-friendly diet. Packing your diet with fruit and veg, fibre-rich foods and lean proteins, will also help you maintain a healthy weight, which will lighten the load on your joints and reduce your risk of type 2 diabetes. Probiotic yoghurts or drinks will help replenish levels of gut bacteria.

Eat yourself younger

Follow our seven-day eating plan for a vital, more radiant you

You've heard the phrase 'beauty comes from within'? Well, it's more than a well-worn adage. Scientists and skincare experts are discovering that we *do* have the ability to feed our skin from within – your diet is as key as your skin cream. They've found a sound approach to eating is one way to help fight the visible signs of ageing. Thankfully, a skin-kind

> ❝ *Eat oily fish, avocados and seeds to help your skin's cells retain water* ❞

diet that hydrates your skin's cells, fights free-radical damage and repairs collagen, is also one that will benefit your health in many other ways. It's based on common-sense principles you can easily adopt. Top of your list should be quality sources of essential fatty acids, such as oily fish; avocados and seeds, to help your skin's cells retain water; lean protein, such as fish, chicken and pulses, which help repair skin cells; antioxidant-rich fruit and veg, such as leafy greens and berries; and two litres of water a day to keep your complexion plump and hydrated.

Beauty nutrients

Here are the top key vitamins and minerals with benefits for your skin – and where to find them.

○ **Vitamin C** is an important antioxidant shown to reduce the free radical damage to your skin caused by sunlight and pollution. Free radicals damage the fibres, such as collagen, that support your skin structure, causing wrinkles and signs of ageing. Vitamin C aids collagen production, which gives skin its firmness and helps it repair itself.
Vitamin C-rich foods: citrus fruits, berries, mangoes, kiwi, red peppers, cabbage.

○ **Beta carotene** is necessary for the maintenance and repair of your skin tissue. Medical studies show it plays an important role in reducing lines and wrinkles.
Vitamin A-rich foods: butternut squash, sweet potatoes, mangoes, carrots, spinach.

○ **Vitamin E** plays an important anti-ageing role for your skin. It has excellent moisturising properties and is shown to help reduce the appearance of wrinkles and fine lines and make your skin look and feel smoother.
Vitamin E-rich foods: wholegrains, avocados, egg yolks, nuts, seeds, spinach, watercress.

○ **Selenium**, a powerful antioxidant, increases your skin's elasticity, helps prevent acne and has been shown to reduce wrinkles and fine lines.
Selenium-rich foods: nuts (especially Brazil nuts), poultry, wholegrains, eggs, beef.

○ **Zinc** is required for the synthesis of collagen and elastin in your skin and works to clear it by controlling oil production. It helps keep your nails and hair healthy.
Zinc-rich foods: wholegrains (oats), shellfish, pumpkin seeds, nuts (almonds and walnuts).

○ **Essential fats** help keep skin cells hydrated, plump and youthful, preventing dry hair and skin. Omega 6 oils can help regulate the skin's oiliness and heal blemishes.
Essential fat-rich foods: oily fish, nuts, seeds.

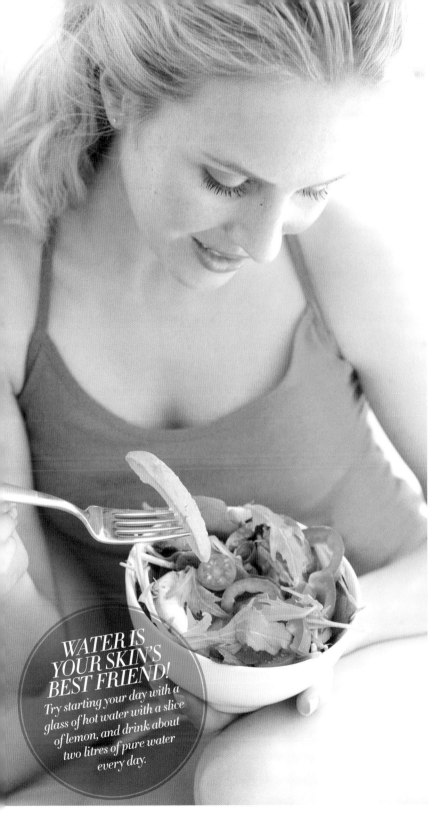

7-DAY LOOK-YOUNGER DIET

Day 1:

BREAKFAST

Berries, yoghurt and pumpkin seeds.

Combine fresh blueberries and raspberries with 120g low-fat live natural yoghurt and some pumpkin seeds.

BENEFIT: Berries are high in vitamin C, which help protect your skin from free radical damage. Pumpkin seeds are high in omega 6 oils to keep your skin moisturised.

SNACK

Fresh gazpacho and almonds

Blend half a cucumber, four tomatoes, half a red pepper, one garlic clove, two spring onions and fresh basil with one tablespoon each of olive oil and red wine vinegar. Sieve and add water to get the consistency you like. Serve cold, topped with flaked almonds.

BENEFIT: Raw veg are packed with antioxidant vitamins and minerals. Almonds are a source of essential fats that help build skin cells and heal blemishes.

LUNCH

Grilled chicken and puy lentil salad

Top baby spinach with 50g cooled puy lentils, grated carrot, lemon juice and 100g free-range chicken.

BENEFIT: Lentils and chicken are a good source of selenium — great for healthy skin and hair.

SNACK

Balsamic strawberries with mascarpone cheese

Marinate 100g strawberries with 1tsp balsamic vinegar and mix in mascarpone with low-fat live natural yoghurt.

BENEFIT: The yoghurt provides your gut with friendly bacteria to aid digestion and boost your skin.

DINNER

Roast salmon with roasted tomatoes

Pre-heat your oven to 180°C/gas mark 4. Place the salmon and tomatoes on a baking tray and roast on the middle shelf for 10-12 minutes until the salmon is just cooked. Serve with basil pesto coated baby potatoes.

BENEFIT: Tomatoes are rich in antioxidants, which help protect against sunburn and cancer. Salmon is a good source of essential fat to help keep your skin supple.

7-DAY **LOOK-YOUNGER** DIET

Day 2:

BREAKFAST
Coconut bircher muesli with mango

Mix 25ml coconut milk with 40g rolled oats, leave to soak and serve with 2tbsp low-fat live natural yoghurt, lime juice and 50g fresh mango.

BENEFIT: Oats are a good source of zinc, which helps control the production of oil in the skin. Coconut milk is rich in copper, which keeps your skin elastic and flexible.

SNACK
Nectarines with ginger

For a delicious snack, eat 100g sliced nectarine with some grated root ginger and a handful of pumpkin seeds.

BENEFIT: Raw seeds eaten like this are a good source of omega 6 essential fat. Omega 6 oils can help regulate the skin's oiliness and heal blemishes.

LUNCH
King prawns with coriander pesto

Mix pesto ingredients in a blender: 30g cashew nuts, 10g coriander, garlic, chilli flakes, sesame oil and some lime juice. Serve with a wild rice salad: cook a blend of wild and brown rice (60g uncooked), mix with spring onions, blanched baby corn, mangetout, red and yellow pepper and some soy sauce and cooked peeled prawns.

BENEFIT: Shellfish are a low-fat, low-calorie source of protein and are full of minerals, including antioxidant selenium, which can protect your skin against ageing.

SNACK
Cashew nut and beetroot pâté

Blend some red pepper, beetroot, cashew nuts and ginger with soy sauce and cider vinegar. Serve with some fresh raw sugar snap peas.

BENEFIT: Beetroot is a good source of fibre and is rich in antioxidants which help boost the immune system. It helps build collagen to keep your cells supple.

DINNER
Marinated beef, chilli and green papaya and Asian coleslaw salad

Combine 100g unripe green papaya, 1tsp each of green chilli, fresh mint and coriander and lemon juice with 50g each of thinly sliced red and white cabbage. Pepper 100g rump steak and cook in oil. Slice thinly and serve with the papaya coleslaw and some rice noodles.

BENEFIT: Cabbage contains antioxidant vitamins A and C, which help prevent sun damage.

Day 3:

BREAKFAST
Smoked salmon and scrambled egg

Prepare 50g smoked salmon with one free range scrambled egg. Serve with roasted baby plum tomatoes, a squeeze of lemon juice and a sprinkle of black pepper.

SKIN BENEFIT: The protein and retinol found in eggs helps collagen production and aids skin regeneration.

SNACK
Cherries and hazelnuts

For a delicious morning snack eat 100g seasonal fresh cherries with a small handful of hazelnuts.

BENEFIT: Cherries are a good source of vitamin C, which will help protect the skin from free radical damage.

LUNCH
Roast chicken superfood salad

Mix salad ingredients: 40g quinoa, 15g alfalfa sprouts, 30g watercress, 30g mange tout and 80g broccoli. Thinly slice 80g skinless roast chicken and 80g roast baby beetroot on top and drizzle with lime juice.

BENEFIT: This salad is packed with super ingredients for the skin. Quinoa is a rich source of perfect protein and is easily digested so it doesn't cause bloating.

SNACK
Sun-dried tomato hummus with sugar snap peas

Blend chickpeas, tahini, garlic and sun-dried tomatoes. Serve with 100g washed, raw sugar snaps and dip into the sun-dried tomato hummus for a healthy snack.

BENEFIT: Tomatoes are rich in vitamins A and C and lycopene, an important antioxidant, which helps defend your skin from free radical damage.

DINNER
Barbecued tuna steak nicoise

Combine 100g green beans, 10g black olives, two ripe tomatoes, two anchovy fillets, 25g hard boiled quail eggs, seasonal salad leaves and 2tbsp extra virgin olive oil. Mix with a red wine and Dijon mustard dressing. Chargrill the red pepper, remove the skin and slice. Barbecue 100g yellow fin tuna steak and place on top of the salad.

BENEFIT: Tuna's omega 3 essential fat content helps your skin's cell walls retain moisture so preventing dry skin.

Day 4:

BREAKFAST
Fresh blackberries, cinnamon spiced apples and live natural yoghurt

Peel and roast one apple with cinnamon (180°C/gas mark 4) for 10 minutes, cool and mix it with organic, probiotic natural yoghurt, berries and cashew nuts.

BENEFIT: Cinnamon aids blood sugar control, helping prevent unhealthy snacking.

SNACK
Babaganoush with crudités

Sauté aubergine cubes until soft in a little olive oil. Transfer them to a food processor and combine with half a clove of garlic, 1tsp cumin, a drizzle of lemon juice and some fresh basil leaves. Serve with 50g raw carrot and 50g cucumber batons.

BENEFIT: Aubergines are a rich source of bioflavonoids – antioxidants that protect against ageing.

LUNCH
Smoked mackerel salad with horseradish dressing

Flake a fillet of naturally smoked mackerel over a salad of mixed leaves, sliced peppers and halved cherry tomatoes. Combine the horseradish sauce with natural yoghurt and drizzle over the salad.

BENEFIT: Mackerel is a good source of vitamin E, which has excellent moisturising properties.

SNACK
Citrus fruit salad with dried apricots and seeds

Mix together segments of 50g each of fresh orange and grapefruit with 20g chopped organic dried apricots and a small handful of black sesame seeds sprinkled on top.

BENEFIT: Citrus fruits are a source of antioxidants, which help build collagen to keep your cells elastic.

DINNER
Stuffed red pepper with goat's cheese

Roast half a red pepper in a pre-heated oven (180°C/gas mark 4) on the middle shelf for 10 minutes. Quarter a tomato and stuff into the pepper with a sliced garlic clove. Roast for 10 minutes. Place a slice of goat's cheese on top and grill on a high heat until it's bubbling. Serve with sautéed spinach and steamed green beans.

BENEFIT: Cheese is rich in vitamin A which helps to maintain skin health.

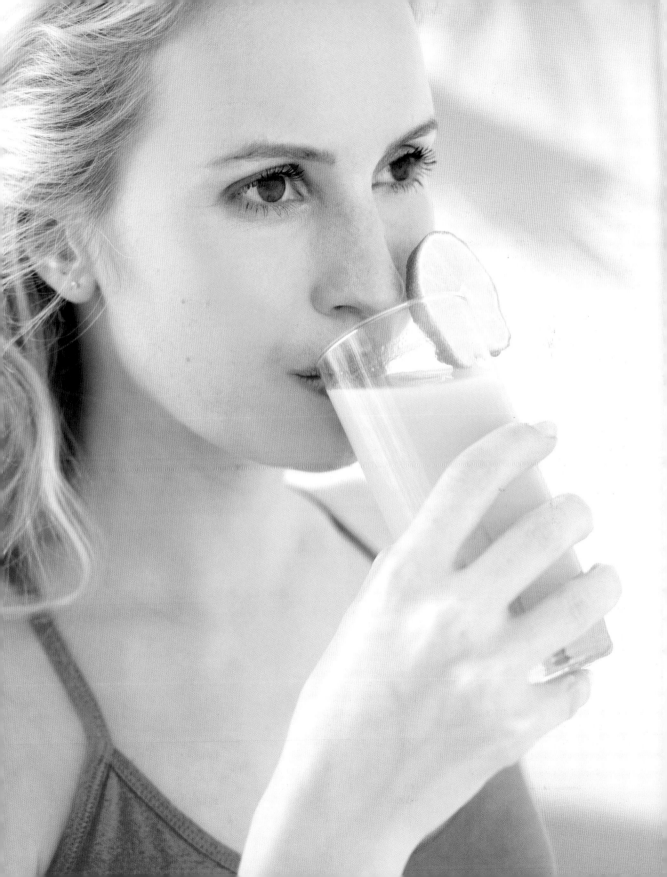

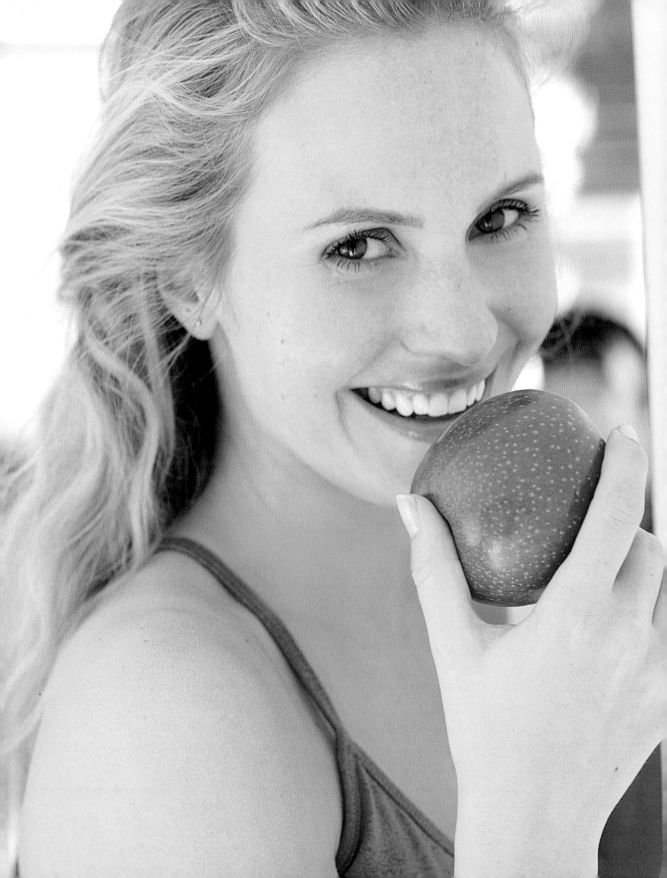

Day 5:

BREAKFAST
Watercress and cherry tomato omelette

Dry fry/roast a small handful of halved cherry tomatoes, add a little olive oil and add one beaten free-range egg loosened with a little milk/water. Add a handful of fresh watercress leaves and finish under the grill to make it soufflé.

BENEFITS: This protein-rich breakfast will sustain you all morning. Watercress is full of the antioxidant betacarotene, vital for protecting you against ageing.

SNACK
100g fresh grapes with a small handful of Brazil nuts

BENEFITS: Grapes are powerful detoxifiers and can improve the condition of your skin.

LUNCH
Tiger prawns served with an orange and mint salsa

Stir fry 80g prawns and cook 40g brown rice. Mix the rice with chopped coriander and serve on a bed of rocket with 50g kidney beans and a juicy orange, apple and mint salsa. Add apple, orange, ginger and mint to a food processor and blend until it's a smooth salsa.

BENEFITS: Prawns are a good source of zinc needed to make collagen and elastin in your skin. Zinc also controls the production of oil in the skin.

SNACK
Spiced poached pears

Lightly poach a chopped pear in water with half a teaspoon of Chinese five-spice and star anise. When tender, take out and serve with 1dsp Greek yoghurt.

BENEFITS: Live natural yoghurt will help provide the gut with friendly bacteria to aid digestion.

DINNER
Balsamic rainbow trout

Pre-heat an oven to 180°C/gas mark 4. Place the fillet of trout on a sheet of foil, drizzle 1tbsp balsamic over it and place a couple of basil leaves on top. Fold up the foil to make an envelope. Place on a baking sheet and roast for eight minutes until the trout is just cooked. Serve with flaked almonds, asparagus and roasted cherry tomatoes.

BENEFITS: Oily fish (eg trout) is a good source of essential fat which helps keep cells hydrated.

Day 6:

BREAKFAST
Strawberry and banana bircher muesli

Blend 40g each of strawberries and bananas with 120g live natural yoghurt. Stir in 30g oats and leave for 30 minutes. Serve with a couple of nuts on top.

BENEFITS Strawberries contain alpha-hydroxyl acid which can help to clear up blemishes.

SNACK
Avocado guacamole

Blend half an avocado with some lime juice, chili and 1 tsp chopped red onion. Add in half a chopped tomato. Serve with two brown rice cakes or some corn chips.

BENEFITS: Avocados are a good source of vitamin E, which has excellent moisturising properties. Eating vegetables raw like this means you receive their maximum nutrient content.

LUNCH
Roasted vegetable and buffalo mozzarella salad

Roast a selection of vegetables (red onion, courgette, peppers and aubergine) in the middle of a pre-heated oven (200°C, gas mark 6). Steam 00g baby potatoes and mix with the roasted veg then top with pieces of buffalo mozzarella cheese (40g). Serve on a bed of rocket leaves with some balsamic vinegar.

BENEFITS: Red peppers are a rich source of betacarotene and vitamin C.

SNACK
Mango and pumpkin seeds

Serve 100g mango with some raw pumpkin seeds.

BENEFITS: Mangoes are rich in vitamin C and betacarotene and are said to cleanse the blood. Seeds are a source of omega 6 essential fat which can help blemishes.

DINNER
Fillet of beef and shitake noodles

Sear a small fillet of steak on a griddle and rest. Slice shitake mushrooms and sauté them lightly in a little soy sauce. Place thin rice noodles in a bowl and pour over boiling water. Leave until cooked. Serve the noodles on a bed of rocket, topped with the thinly sliced fillet steak, mushrooms and some chopped cashew nuts, chilli and coriander.

BENEFITS: Mushrooms have immune-boosting and antioxidant properties and can reduce inflammation, helping your skin to look healthier.

Day 7:

BREAKFAST
Grapefruit, rye bread and nut spread

Toast a couple of slices of rye bread. Thinly smooth a natural nut spread on top (we like Carleys Organic Rainforest Nut Butter, £3.89 for 170g, www.natural grocery.co.uk), and serve with 100g grapefruit pieces.

BENEFITS: Rye is a useful source of fibre, needed to maintain a healthy liver, which helps your skin.

SNACK
Kiwi and black sesame seeds

Peel and slice two kiwi fruit and serve with a sprinkling of black sesame seeds.

BENEFITS: Kiwi fruit are a rich source of vitamin C.

LUNCH
Tabbouleh salad with grilled chicken

Drizzle a free range chicken breast in lemon juice, season with black pepper and grill until cooked through. Rest. Wash half a cup of barley couscous, add half a cup of boiling water, cover and leave for 10 minutes. Cool slightly, mix with one and a half cups of chopped parsley, chopped tomatoes, peppers, cucumber, juice of half a lemon and olive oil. Slice the chicken and serve.

BENEFITS: Barley couscous is an excellent source of iron and rich in minerals. Parsley is a powerful diuretic.

SNACK
Hot tomato salsa with crudités

Sauté a handful of halved cherry tomatoes until softened. Cool. Blend with lime juice and fresh coriander, until mixed but still chunky. Add red chilli to the mixture if desired. Serve with celery and sugar snaps.

BENEFITS: Tomatoes are a rich source of the anti-oxidant lycopene and vitamin E, which protects your skin cells from ultra violet light and free radical damage.

DINNER
Feta and pumpkin seed stuffed butternut squash

Halve a small butternut squash and scoop out the seeds and stringy bits. Place in a pre-heated oven (200°C/gas mark 6) on a baking sheet for 30 minutes. Sauté an onion until soft, mix with a few sundried tomatoes, feta cheese, pumpkin seeds and basil. Place the mix into the centre of the cooked butternut. Pop in the oven for 10 minutes and serve with a mixed balsamic dressed salad.

BENEFITS: Butternut squash is rich in betacarotene which helps fight signs of ageing.

Stay-young recipes

Look and feel your best with these anti-ageing dishes

COLD-PRESSED HEMP OIL
Contains omega 3, 6 and 9 fatty acids which keep your heart, skin and hair healthy.

TOFU
A rich source of low-fat protein and a good source of iron.

Marinated tofu and pomegranate salad

Full of anti-ageing antioxidants, this salad is quick to make and is the ideal lunch or starter.

Preparation time: 10 minutes
Serves: 2, or 4 as a starter

Method

O Add 200g mixed leaves to a bowl, sprinkle with a 160g pack of marinated tofu pieces, 100g pomegranate seeds and 1tbsp pumpkin seeds.

O Add the grated zest and juice of an orange and a drizzle of cold-pressed hemp oil.

POMEGRANATES
Packed with antioxidants and high in fibre.

Sweet pepper and spring onion omelette

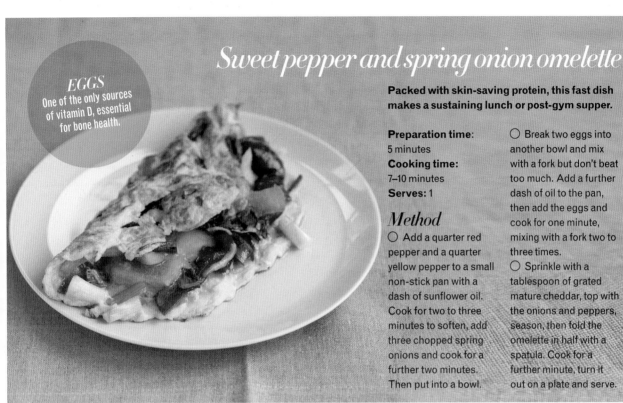

Packed with skin-saving protein, this fast dish makes a sustaining lunch or post-gym supper.

Preparation time: 5 minutes
Cooking time: 7–10 minutes
Serves: 1

Method

○ Add a quarter red pepper and a quarter yellow pepper to a small non-stick pan with a dash of sunflower oil. Cook for two to three minutes to soften, add three chopped spring onions and cook for a further two minutes. Then put into a bowl.

○ Break two eggs into another bowl and mix with a fork but don't beat too much. Add a further dash of oil to the pan, then add the eggs and cook for one minute, mixing with a fork two to three times.

○ Sprinkle with a tablespoon of grated mature cheddar, top with the onions and peppers, season, then fold the omelette in half with a spatula. Cook for a further minute, turn it out on a plate and serve.

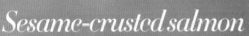

Sesame-crusted salmon

Rich in protein and omega 3s, the perfect beauty foods, this salmon supper is a facelift on a plate!

Preparation time: 10 minutes
Cooking time: 15 minutes
Serves: 2

Method

○ Coat two salmon steaks (120g each approx) with the juice of half a lemon, put on a plate and sprinkle with 2tbsp sesame seeds, making sure they're well coated. Place on a lightly oiled baking sheet, sprinkle any remaining seeds on top and bake in a pre-heated oven 180°C/gas mark 4 for 12–15 minutes.

○ While the salmon cooks, add a 300g bag of stir-fry vegetables (try one with soya beans) to a pan with a dash of toasted sesame oil and a small dash of sunflower oil and cook for 3–5 minutes over a high heat.

○ Place the vegetables on a dish, break the salmon into chunks and arrange on top, then drizzle with 1dsp soy sauce and squeeze of lemon juice.

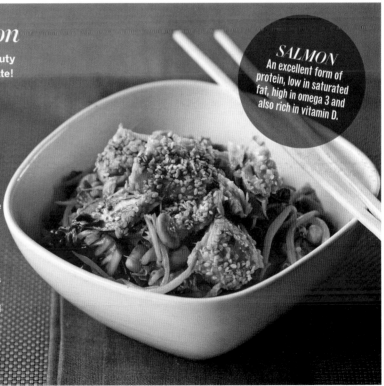

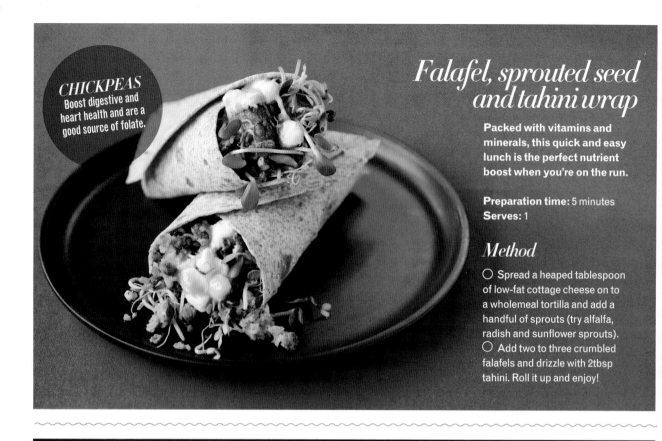

Falafel, sprouted seed and tahini wrap

Packed with vitamins and minerals, this quick and easy lunch is the perfect nutrient boost when you're on the run.

Preparation time: 5 minutes
Serves: 1

Method

○ Spread a heaped tablespoon of low-fat cottage cheese on to a wholemeal tortilla and add a handful of sprouts (try alfalfa, radish and sunflower sprouts).
○ Add two to three crumbled falafels and drizzle with 2tbsp tahini. Roll it up and enjoy!

Quinoa, apricot, lemon and sunflower seeds pilaf

This quinoa pilaf makes an excellent side dish and is also ideal to take to work for lunch.

Preparation time: 10 minutes
Cooking time: 20 minutes
Serves: 4

Method

○ Add a dash of sunflower oil to a saucepan with a finely chopped onion, stir regularly for 3 minutes. Now add a chopped leek, 2 heaped tsp ground cumin, 1 level tsp chilli flakes, a good pinch of salt, 175g quinoa and 500ml boiling water, mix well, cover and simmer gently for 15 minutes.
○ Meanwhile, chop 75g dried apricots and mix with 2 tbsp sunflower seeds and 50g chopped coriander, the juice and grated zest of an unwaxed lemon and 1 tbsp of extra virgin olive oil.
○ When the quinoa is cooked, fluff with a fork and mix with the apricot mixture.

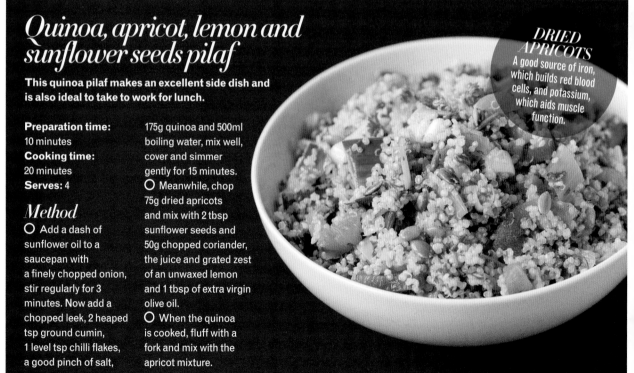

Superfood sandwich

A few nutrient-packed ingredients can turn an ordinary sandwich into a power-packed lunch.

Preparation time: 10 minutes
Serves: 2

Method

○ Spread four slices of wholegrain seeded bread with 1tbsp tahini.

○ Mix a 213g can of sockeye salmon with the juice of half a lemon, 1tbsp live natural yoghurt and some black pepper.

○ Divide the salmon, 75g of alfalfa and radish sprouts, and half a thinly-sliced red pepper to make two sandwiches.

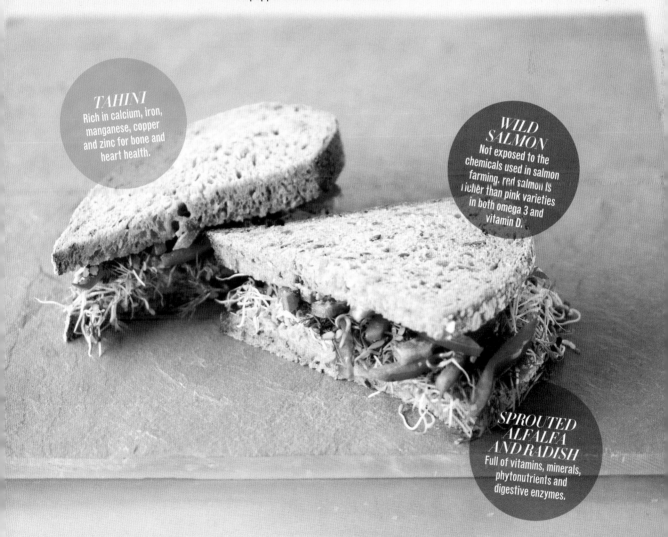

TAHINI
Rich in calcium, iron, manganese, copper and zinc for bone and heart health.

WILD SALMON
Not exposed to the chemicals used in salmon farming, red salmon is richer than pink varieties in both omega 3 and vitamin D.

SPROUTED ALFALFA AND RADISH
Full of vitamins, minerals, phytonutrients and digestive enzymes.

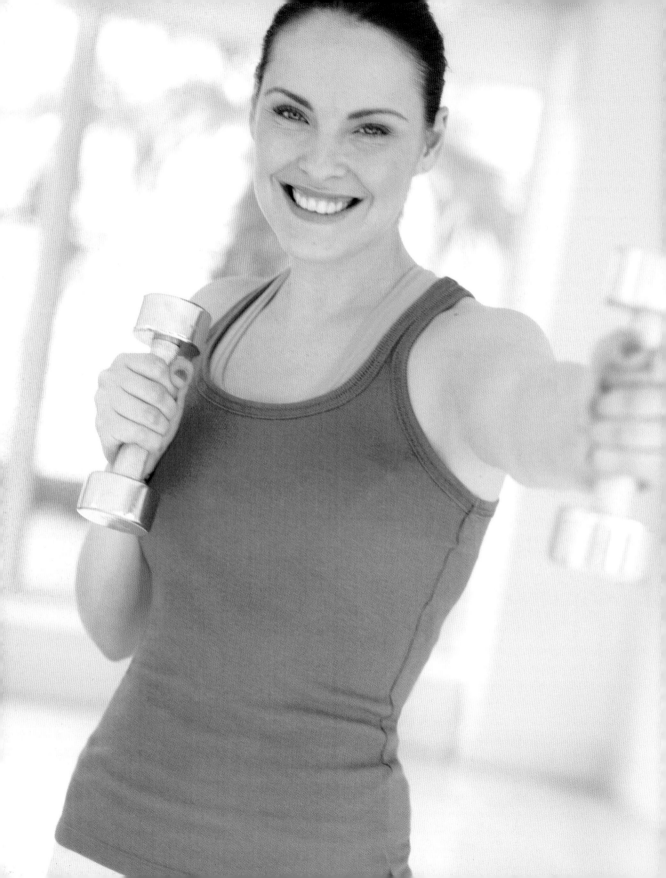

Age-defying exercise

Regular exercise is important for defending your body against ageing. It protects your major organs, gives you energy and helps you maintain a healthy weight. It's also linked to a lower risk of age-related illness, including dementia, osteoporosis, diabetes and heart disease. In this chapter, discover the best workouts to hold back the years.

Age-fighting fit

Regular exercise won't just keep you toned and energised,
the latest research shows it keeps your body young too

There's nothing more youthful than the radiant glow you get after exercising. And research proves that staying active has anti-ageing benefits from top to toe.

IT AGE-PROOFS YOUR CELLS
Exercise keeps you young from the inside out. A study at Saarland University in Germany found that exercise hinders the shortening of telomeres – the protective caps on the ends of all our chromosomes. Telomeres are similar to the plastic tips on the end of shoelaces that stop them unravelling. As telomeres shorten, a cell becomes more susceptible to dying. The researchers also suggest a sedentary lifestyle can make you more susceptible to free-radical damage and inflammation at a cellular level.

IT PROTECTS YOUR HEART
Exercise has rich and multi-layered benefits for your heart, lowering body fat, blood pressure and risk of diabetes, as well as raising levels of heart-protective HDL cholesterol.

IT'S DE-STRESSING
Experts at the University of Missouri-Columbia in the US have found relatively high-intensity exercise is one of the best tools we have for reducing stress and anxiety. And all the better if you exercise outdoors – a study at the University of Essex shows that a five-minute burst of outdoor activity will lift your mood.

IT HELPS AGE-ERASE YOUR SKIN
When you exercise, you increase your circulation and get the blood flowing

> **66** *Regular exercise can slash your risk of breast and colon cancers* **99**

around your body so that it brings nutrients and oxygen to your skin – and a wonderful rosy glow.

IT BOOSTS YOUR BRAIN CELLS
Countless studies show that regular exercise, such as running, can help create new brain cells. It can also significantly lower your risk of age-related brain decline and dementia.

IT CUTS YOUR CANCER RISK
Regular exercise can slash your risk of breast cancer, confirms a study of 74,000 women at the Fred Hutchinson Cancer Research Center in Seattle. And a US review of 52 studies has found it can cut risk of colon cancer by up to 24 per cent.

IT KEEPS YOUR BONES YOUNG
Many factors contribute to bone density, but physical activity is one of the most powerful and proactive ways of maintaining a healthy bone mass. The best bone-stimulating activity is weight-bearing exercise, such as running, walking and weight training. Keeping fit can also help you avoid the loss of flexibility that can come with age.

IT BALANCES YOUR HORMONES
As well as helping minimise PMS symptoms, a study published in the journal *Medicine & Science in Sports & Exercise* shows that if you remain active up to and during the menopause, you can ease common symptoms including anxiety, depression and stress.

IT'S NEVER TOO LATE...
Regular exercising is essential from a young age, but it's such a powerful anti-ageing weapon you'll still get the benefits if you start later. A study by Boston's Brigham and Women's Hospital in the US showed that even taking up exercise after the age of 70, along with eating healthily and not smoking, can boost your life expectancy by 50 per cent.

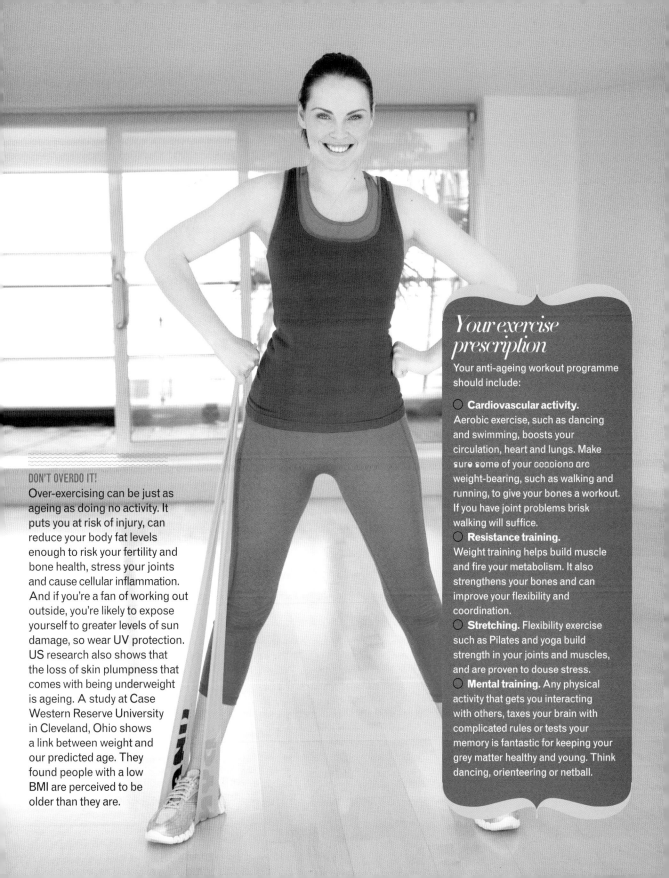

DON'T OVERDO IT!

Over-exercising can be just as ageing as doing no activity. It puts you at risk of injury, can reduce your body fat levels enough to risk your fertility and bone health, stress your joints and cause cellular inflammation. And if you're a fan of working out outside, you're likely to expose yourself to greater levels of sun damage, so wear UV protection. US research also shows that the loss of skin plumpness that comes with being underweight is ageing. A study at Case Western Reserve University in Cleveland, Ohio shows a link between weight and our predicted age. They found people with a low BMI are perceived to be older than they are.

Your exercise prescription

Your anti-ageing workout programme should include:

○ **Cardiovascular activity.** Aerobic exercise, such as dancing and swimming, boosts your circulation, heart and lungs. Make sure some of your sessions are weight-bearing, such as walking and running, to give your bones a workout. If you have joint problems brisk walking will suffice.

○ **Resistance training.** Weight training helps build muscle and fire your metabolism. It also strengthens your bones and can improve your flexibility and coordination.

○ **Stretching.** Flexibility exercise such as Pilates and yoga build strength in your joints and muscles, and are proven to douse stress.

○ **Mental training.** Any physical activity that gets you interacting with others, taxes your brain with complicated rules or tests your memory is fantastic for keeping your grey matter healthy and young. Think dancing, orienteering or netball.

Wonder workouts

We've cherry-picked the most effective forms of exercise
to help you keep those tell-tale signs of ageing at bay

All exercise is anti-ageing, but choose carefully and you can target the areas of your body and health you're most concerned about to stay fit and youthful. From your bones and heart to your pelvic floor, every workout has different benefits.

WALKING

Accessible, thrifty and super-effective – walking is the ultimate anti-ageing exercise. Regular walking is linked to lower risk of heart disease, diabetes, high blood pressure and osteoporosis. But don't dawdle – experts believe that your speed might help you monitor how healthy you are. A study at the University of Pittsburgh in the US found that a person with a walking speed slower than 0.6m per second may be at increased risk of poor health.

RUNNING

It's good for your heart, but running is also a form of weight-bearing exercise, meaning it challenges and strengthens your skeleton. A 21-year study at Stanford University in the US showed runners have fewer disabilities, stay active for longer and halve their risk of an early death.

YOGA

Yoga is a true mind-body experience. It offers a resistance workout, enhancing muscle strength and flexibility, and can help offset lower back pain, stiff joints and loss of balance. But yoga is also an effective stress reliever – in an analysis of its effect on the brain chemical GABA, researchers from Boston University School of Medicine in the US found it's superior to other exercise in terms of its positive effect on mood and anxiety.

PILATES

Pilates' strengthens the core muscles that protect your spine – but it also

> **❝ Researchers have found hitting the dance floor helps you ward off dementia ❞**

enhances joint flexibility, balance and coordination. Crucially, it's great for injury rehabilitation and is gentle enough to be continued into old age. According to a study of 60 women over the age of 65 published in the *Journal of Sports Science and Medicine*, a sustained programme can enhance mobility.

DANCING

Dancing is a weight-bearing form of aerobic exercise and can rev up your grey matter too. Researchers at Albert Einstein College of Medicine in New York found that alongside playing musical instruments, reading and playing board games, hitting the dance floor helps you ward off dementia. Try high-octane Zumba if ballroom is too sedate for you!

SWIMMING

An excellent aerobic workout, great for muscle tone and joint mobility, swimming is kind on an ageing body as your weight is fully supported. Research at Indiana University in the US found that regular and moderately intensive swimming can halt the downward decline of your key age markers, blood pressure, muscle mass, blood chemistry and pulmonary function.

PELVIC FLOOR EXERCISES

It's said that around four million British women have stress incontinence. It occurs when the sphincter muscle isn't strong enough to withstand bladder pressure, and is common after childbirth and pregnancy. One preventative step is to shape up your pelvic floor muscles, which wrap from the front of your pelvis to your tailbone and keep all your internal organs in place. Daily Kegel exercises are a must. Sit on the arm of a chair with your legs slightly apart then contract your muscles around your urethra, vagina and rectum as if trying to stop yourself peeing. Don't strain, hold, then relax. Do 10 reps of 10 seconds every day.

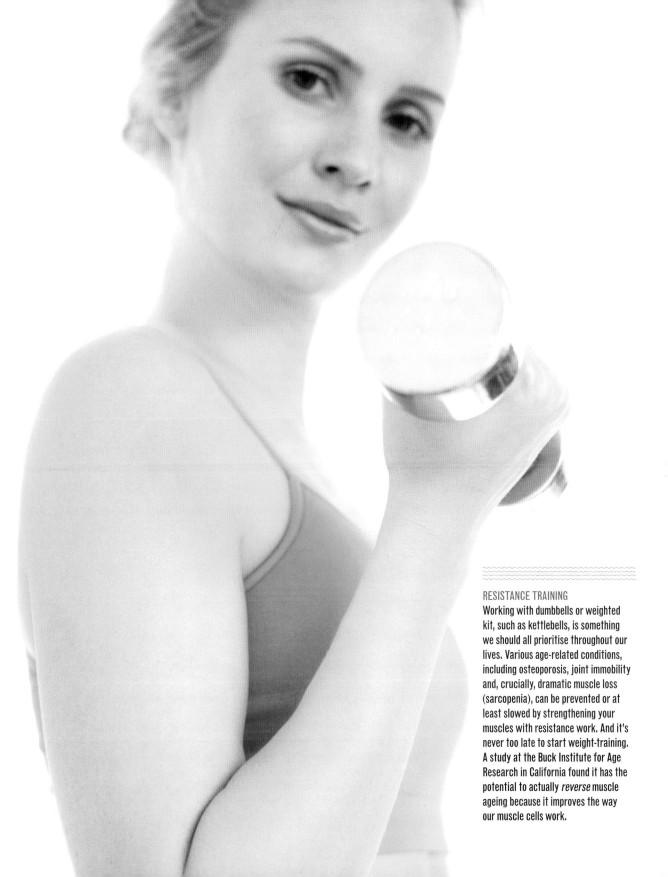

RESISTANCE TRAINING

Working with dumbbells or weighted kit, such as kettlebells, is something we should all prioritise throughout our lives. Various age-related conditions, including osteoporosis, joint immobility and, crucially, dramatic muscle loss (sarcopenia), can be prevented or at least slowed by strengthening your muscles with resistance work. And it's never too late to start weight-training. A study at the Buck Institute for Age Research in California found it has the potential to actually *reverse* muscle ageing because it improves the way our muscle cells work.

Act your age

Tailor your exercise programme to suit your age, and keep your youthful glow

In our childhood it was leapfrog, in our teens cross country or athletics. But too often, as we reach adulthood, our activity levels decline – just when our bodies really need exercise. While high-impact aerobics or running may not be your thing, there's a workout that's just right for you and your body's needs. From bone-building resistance workouts to rejuvenating yoga, finding the right workout for your age can help you stay fit, strong and slim through the years.

Time to build your cardio health and bone strength.
You're at the peak of your fitness in your 20s, and as your body is still building up bone mass, maximise your reserves by working out regularly, especially with weight-bearing exercise. Although the body's natural drop in aerobic fitness (10 per cent a decade) starts in your 20s, you can cut this by as much as 50 per cent by exercising. It's likely you'll be bursting with natural energy, but if you find it hard to motivate yourself, try group or competitive sports, such as netball, tennis and hockey – or something upbeat such as dancing, so you can feed off the enthusiasm of others. Studies also show that exercise will also help you manage PMS-related symptoms including mood swings and abdominal cramps.

Boost your lean muscle mass to up your metabolism.
Your 30s are often very demanding, with work and family needs vying for your attention. Staying fit will help you cope with this busy decade as well as ward of the health challenges of the next. Now's the time to ratchet up your resistance exercise. This will help you defy the natural decline in muscle, boosting your metabolic rate and helping

> *If you're squeezed for time start doing active commuting by walking or cycling to work*

keep your weight in check. Remember your muscles adapt quickly, so ramp up your programme every six to eight weeks, by using heavier weights or increasing your reps. Age-related muscle loss is greater in your lower body than your upper so make sure your programme is balanced. Pregnancy, and long-term habits such as working in an office or carrying a heavy bag can have an impact on your back and flexibility, so make time for a weekly Pilates or yoga class. If your work and family commitments mean you're squeezed for time, try high-impact short circuits, start active commuting by walking or cycling to work or explore home workouts.

Prevent middle-age spread with high-impact and endurance workouts.
Just because you've hit the big four-O, it doesn't mean your fitness will decline. Simply carry on looking after your body and keep challenging yourself. Adapt your resistance programme regularly to increase the demand on your muscles, and ditto your aerobic programme. Studies show you can maintain your VO_2 max – your aerobic capacity – with endurance training. Any activity that requires staying power will do. For a challenge, enter a long-distance running event. Besides the physical benefits, having something to focus on will fire your motivation levels, especially if you're raising funds for charity. Or try a triathlon – the combination of running, with low-impact swimming and cycling is much kinder on joints than pure running. Prioritise weight-bearing exercise – as you approach the menopause and the dip in your bone-protective hormone oestrogen, this is the time accrue some

strength. But don't overdo things. Your body is less forgiving in your 40s than in your 20s, so take a steady approach to training and ask a professional for guidance if necessary.

Keep your heart healthy with regular aerobic exercise – but be kind to yourself!
Don't be misled into thinking it's all downhill from here. More than half a million Brits over 50 have run a marathon. The key now is to be conscious of your health and fitness on a daily basis and follow a structured exercise plan to combat age-related conditions. The biggie this decade is the menopause, so take action to prevent deep visceral fat from settling around your waistline. It can narrow your arteries and raise cholesterol, and increase your risk of type 2 diabetes, high blood pressure and dementia. It's also a risk factor for breast and colon cancers.

But tummy fat is not inevitable. Reduce fat levels all over with a sustained aerobic and resistance programme. If you're worried about your joints, focus on low-impact aerobic exercise such as walking, cycling and swimming. Using a Step is particularly good – it combines cardio and strength exercise but, because you're moving against gravity, pressure on your joints is minimised. To lift your mood and ease stress, try a sociable form of exercise, such as dancing. Or try tai chi, it's great for balance, coordination, building bone mass and, according to researchers at the University of California, Los Angeles, can ease depression.

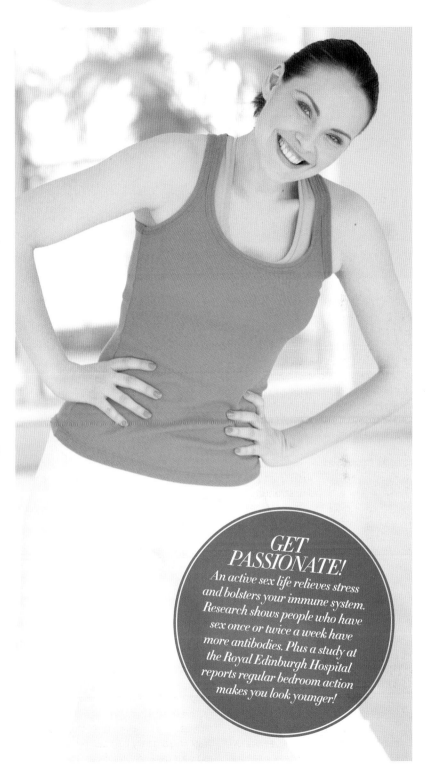

GET PASSIONATE!
An active sex life relieves stress and bolsters your immune system. Research shows people who have sex once or twice a week have more antibodies. Plus a study at the Royal Edinburgh Hospital reports regular bedroom action makes you look younger!

Anti-ageing workout

Tone up your trouble zones, and watch the years melt away with this age-defying exercise plan

This workout has been devised to help you banish bingo wings and muffin tops for good – all those stubborn areas that stop you feeling svelte and youthful. The exercises have the added benefit of being weight-bearing, so they'll also help boost your bone density.

❝ Wear a supportive bra, good trainers and a sweat-wicking tee when you work out. ❞

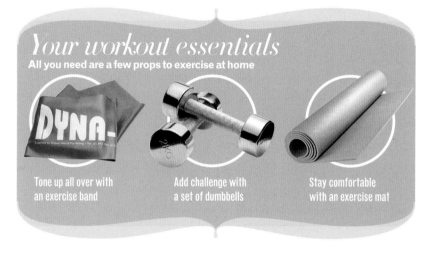

Your workout essentials
All you need are a few props to exercise at home

Tone up all over with an exercise band

Add challenge with a set of dumbbells

Stay comfortable with an exercise mat

To get maximum benefits, add impact exercises, such as walking, running or aerobics where both feet are not in contact with the floor at the same time. Run to boost both your bone density and energy or use a Step to get a high-impact workout.

Before you begin...

This quick plan only takes 30 minutes, providing you practise it three times a week. For better results, gradually make the workout more intense by adding more weight, extra reps or both, week

by week. If you do your cardio before the exercises, your performance will be significantly better, as your muscles will be warm, making you more flexible.

○ **Look the part** To safeguard your wellbeing, wear the right gear – that means a supportive bra, sports-specific socks, good trainers, sweat-wicking tee and snug capri pants, shorts or leggings.

○ **Get kitted up** If you're working out at home, buying some essential kit can elevate your workout to a new level. Aside from an exercise mat, think about getting a set of dumbbells, ankle and wrist

weights, gym ball – the added wobble will engage your stabilising muscles – and Dyna-Band or similar resistance band.

○ **Stay safe** Always warm up to prepare your muscles and joints – and engage your core muscles to protect your back. Perform each exercise with precision but don't get carried away. Don't exercise if you're unwell, stop immediately if you feel pain and progress your workouts incrementally. Post workout, elongate your muscles and flush out lactic acid to prevent soreness by stretching for at least five minutes.

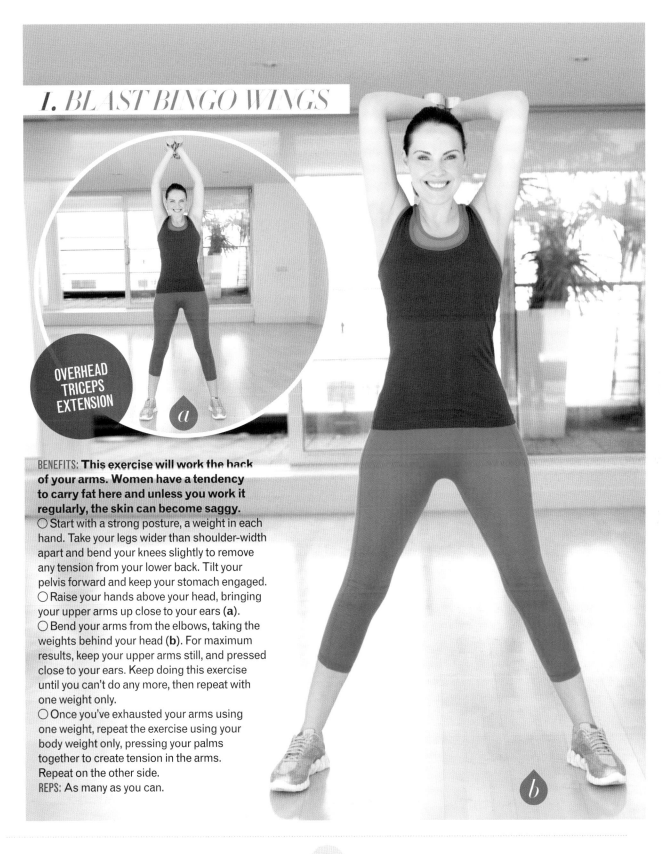

1. BLAST BINGO WINGS

OVERHEAD TRICEPS EXTENSION

a

BENEFITS: This exercise will work the back of your arms. Women have a tendency to carry fat here and unless you work it regularly, the skin can become saggy.

○ Start with a strong posture, a weight in each hand. Take your legs wider than shoulder-width apart and bend your knees slightly to remove any tension from your lower back. Tilt your pelvis forward and keep your stomach engaged.

○ Raise your hands above your head, bringing your upper arms up close to your ears (**a**).

○ Bend your arms from the elbows, taking the weights behind your head (**b**). For maximum results, keep your upper arms still, and pressed close to your ears. Keep doing this exercise until you can't do any more, then repeat with one weight only.

○ Once you've exhausted your arms using one weight, repeat the exercise using your body weight only, pressing your palms together to create tension in the arms. Repeat on the other side.

REPS: As many as you can.

b

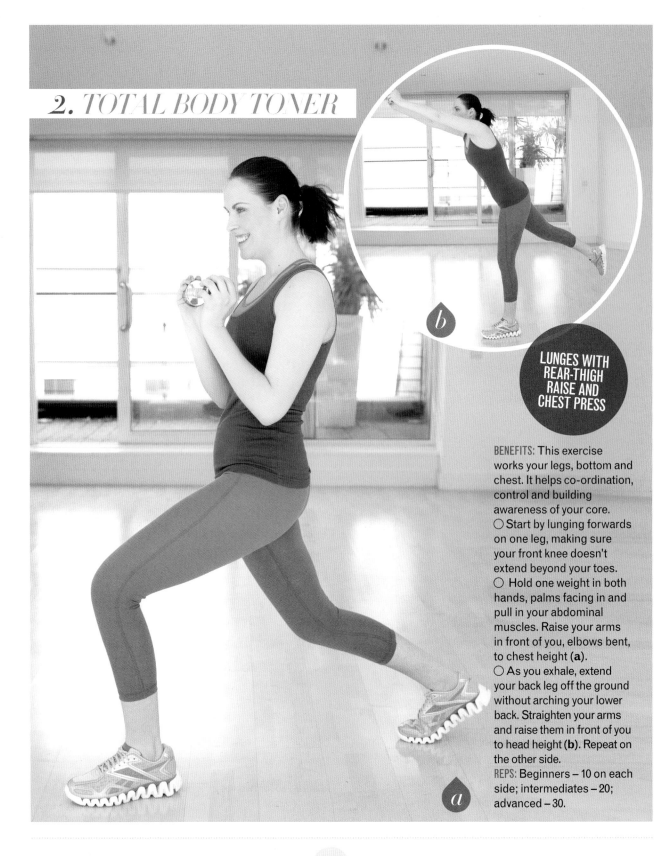

2. TOTAL BODY TONER

LUNGES WITH REAR-THIGH RAISE AND CHEST PRESS

BENEFITS: This exercise works your legs, bottom and chest. It helps co-ordination, control and building awareness of your core.
○ Start by lunging forwards on one leg, making sure your front knee doesn't extend beyond your toes.
○ Hold one weight in both hands, palms facing in and pull in your abdominal muscles. Raise your arms in front of you, elbows bent, to chest height (**a**).
○ As you exhale, extend your back leg off the ground without arching your lower back. Straighten your arms and raise them in front of you to head height (**b**). Repeat on the other side.
REPS: Beginners – 10 on each side; intermediates – 20; advanced – 30.

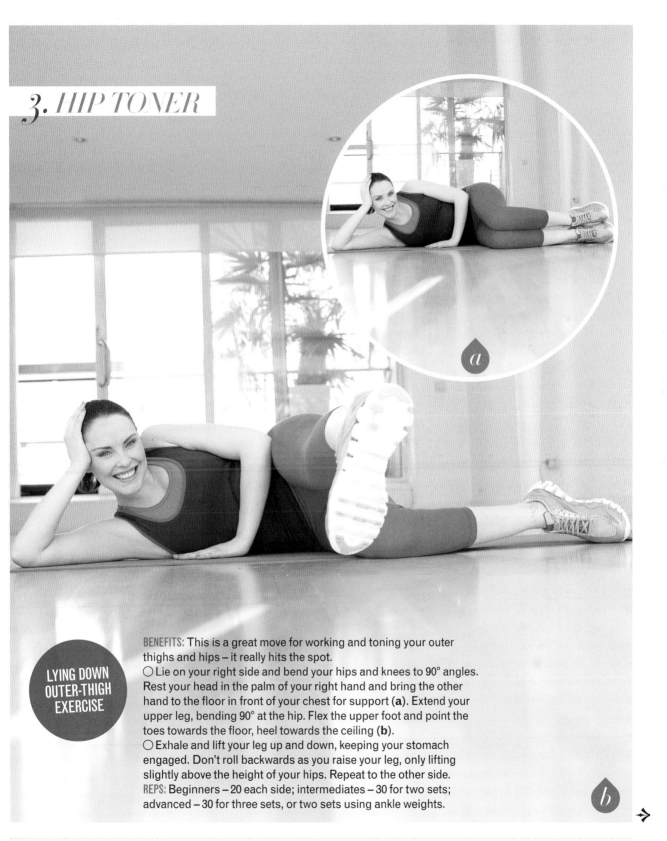

3. HIP TONER

LYING DOWN OUTER-THIGH EXERCISE

BENEFITS: This is a great move for working and toning your outer thighs and hips – it really hits the spot.

○ Lie on your right side and bend your hips and knees to 90° angles. Rest your head in the palm of your right hand and bring the other hand to the floor in front of your chest for support (**a**). Extend your upper leg, bending 90° at the hip. Flex the upper foot and point the toes towards the floor, heel towards the ceiling (**b**).

○ Exhale and lift your leg up and down, keeping your stomach engaged. Don't roll backwards as you raise your leg, only lifting slightly above the height of your hips. Repeat to the other side.

REPS: Beginners – 20 each side; intermediates – 30 for two sets; advanced – 30 for three sets, or two sets using ankle weights.

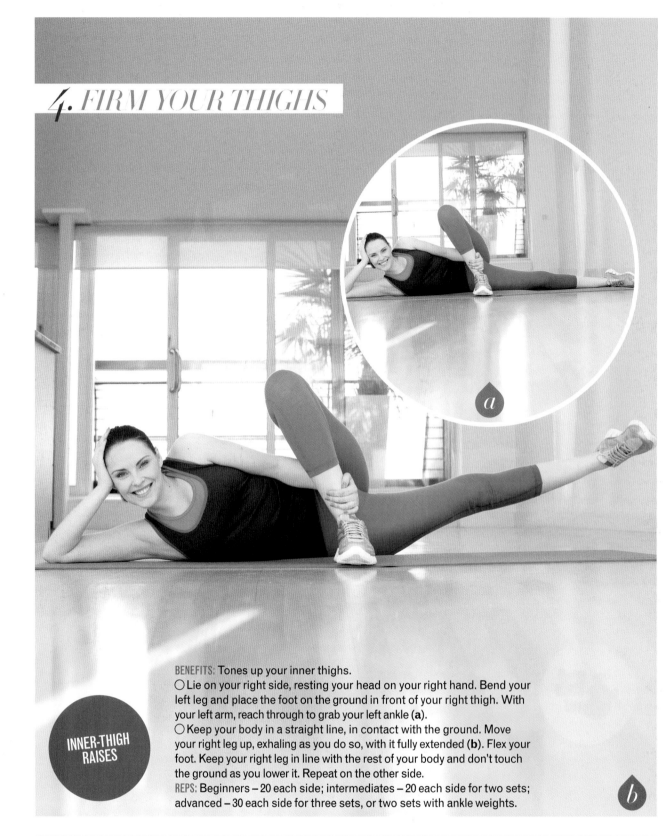

4. FIRM YOUR THIGHS

INNER-THIGH RAISES

BENEFITS: Tones up your inner thighs.

○ Lie on your right side, resting your head on your right hand. Bend your left leg and place the foot on the ground in front of your right thigh. With your left arm, reach through to grab your left ankle (**a**).

○ Keep your body in a straight line, in contact with the ground. Move your right leg up, exhaling as you do so, with it fully extended (**b**). Flex your foot. Keep your right leg in line with the rest of your body and don't touch the ground as you lower it. Repeat on the other side.

REPS: Beginners – 20 each side; intermediates – 20 each side for two sets; advanced – 30 each side for three sets, or two sets with ankle weights.

5. BOOST YOUR BUST

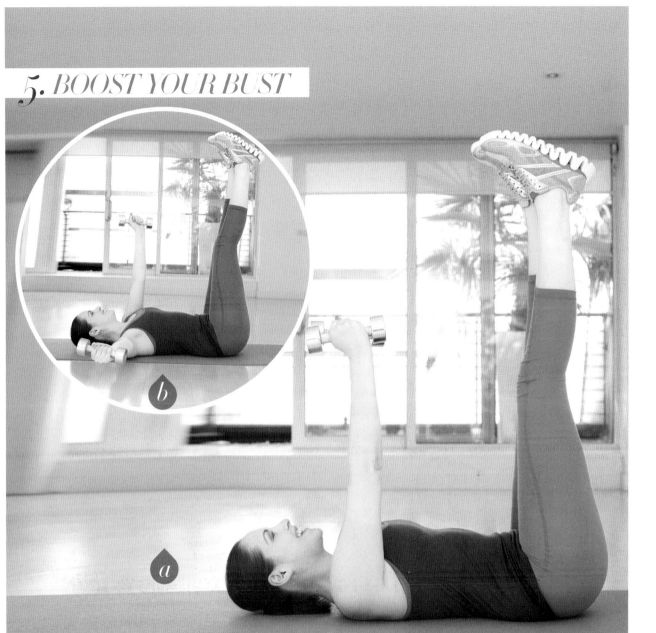

LYING DOWN SINGLE ARM CHEST FLYES

BENEFITS: This is a great stabiliser for activating your core and working your chest muscles.
○ Lying on your back, bring both legs straight up in the air. Draw your navel to your spine and press your lower back into the floor. Flex your feet and keep your legs straight. Raise your arms so your hands are straight above your shoulders **(a)**. Take your arms out to the sides, with your elbows slightly bent. Return to the start position.
○ Advanced version. Extend your legs further away from your body to increase the challenge to your core muscles. Taking one arm to the floor, slightly bend the elbow, without the arm touching the floor **(b)**. Repeat with the other arm.
REPS: Beginners – 10 each side for two sets; intermediates and advanced – 20 each side for two sets.

6. TONE UP YOUR BOTTOM

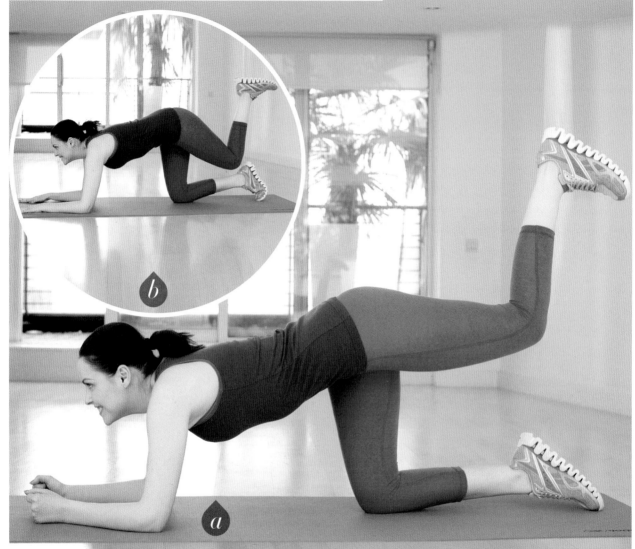

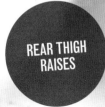

REAR THIGH RAISES

BENEFITS: This is a great exercise for building a high, perky bottom and hopefully keeping it there. It's also a great core exercise.

○ Start on all-fours, toes curled under and resting on your forearms. Raise one leg, letting your heel lead the way and with the sole of your foot facing the ceiling (**a**).

○ Keep your elbows under your chest and avoid leaning too far forwards. Keep your stomach engaged and maintain a neutral spine. Lower your knee to the opposite heel, keeping the rest of the body still as you do so (**b**).

REPS: Beginners – 20 each side; intermediates – 20 each side for two sets; advanced – 30 each side for three sets, or two sets using ankle weights.

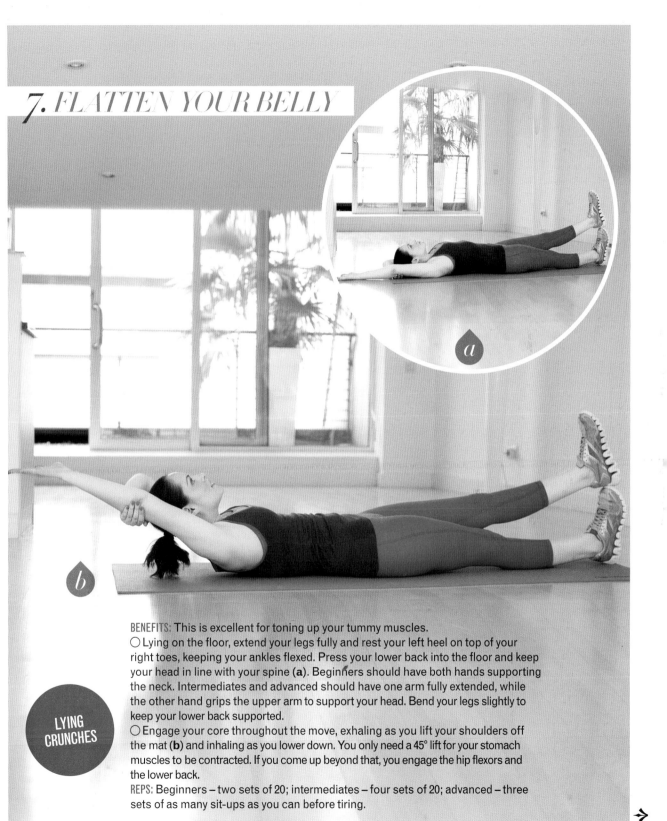

7. FLATTEN YOUR BELLY

LYING CRUNCHES

BENEFITS: This is excellent for toning up your tummy muscles.

○ Lying on the floor, extend your legs fully and rest your left heel on top of your right toes, keeping your ankles flexed. Press your lower back into the floor and keep your head in line with your spine (**a**). Beginners should have both hands supporting the neck. Intermediates and advanced should have one arm fully extended, while the other hand grips the upper arm to support your head. Bend your legs slightly to keep your lower back supported.

○ Engage your core throughout the move, exhaling as you lift your shoulders off the mat (**b**) and inhaling as you lower down. You only need a 45° lift for your stomach muscles to be contracted. If you come up beyond that, you engage the hip flexors and the lower back.

REPS: Beginners – two sets of 20; intermediates – four sets of 20; advanced – three sets of as many sit-ups as you can before tiring.

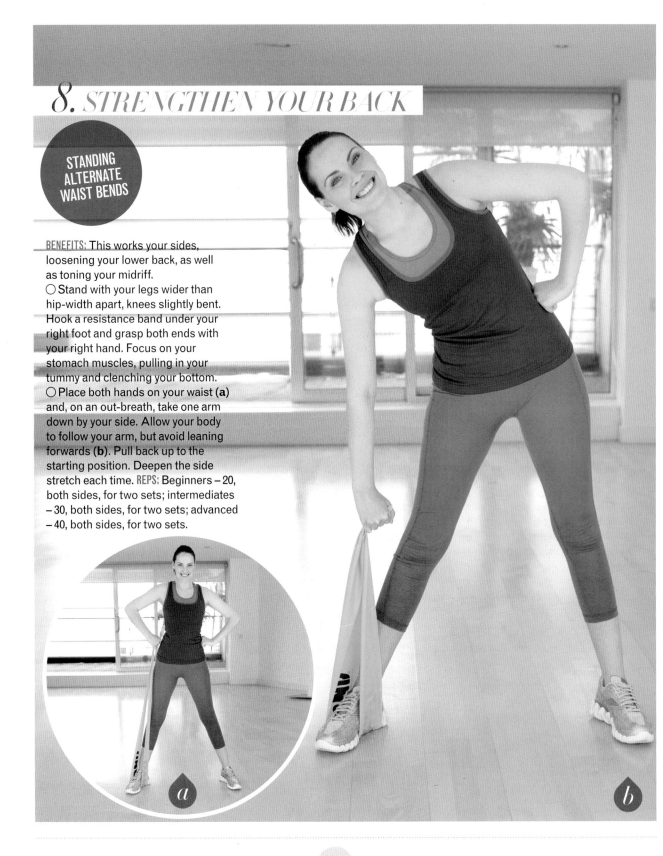

8. STRENGTHEN YOUR BACK

STANDING ALTERNATE WAIST BENDS

BENEFITS: This works your sides, loosening your lower back, as well as toning your midriff.

○ Stand with your legs wider than hip-width apart, knees slightly bent. Hook a resistance band under your right foot and grasp both ends with your right hand. Focus on your stomach muscles, pulling in your tummy and clenching your bottom.

○ Place both hands on your waist (**a**) and, on an out-breath, take one arm down by your side. Allow your body to follow your arm, but avoid leaning forwards (**b**). Pull back up to the starting position. Deepen the side stretch each time. REPS: Beginners – 20, both sides, for two sets; intermediates – 30, both sides, for two sets; advanced – 40, both sides, for two sets.

a

b

Resist those signs of ageing!

Exercising every day will not only give you a younger looking, toned body, but your skin, posture and energy levels will benefit too

One of the easiest ways to tone and strengthen major muscle groups is by using a Dyna-Band®. This resistance band is ideal for home use and will tone, strengthen and define your arms, shoulders, waist, tummy, back, buttocks and legs.

In fact, nearly every exercise you can do in the gym can be done in the privacy of your own home. Unlike free weights and machines, which create tension in just one direction, the bands give you resistance both ways (tightening and releasing it). You'll benefit from 'concentric' contraction, which causes muscles to shorten, and 'eccentric' contraction, which elongates muscles and sculpts your body.

You can control the tension of the Dyna-Band® to work different muscle groups, adjust the level of difficulty and add variety to your fitness plan.

Strength training exercises using the Dyna-Band® will help increase lean muscle mass and counteract the loss of muscle mass associated with ageing. Benefits of increased muscle mass are:

○ **Increased resting metabolic rate**. The more muscle you have, the more calories your body will burn, even at rest.

○ **Increased bone density**. Muscle exerts twisting forces on your bones, causing them to become stronger and more dense and helping prevent osteoporosis.

○ **Blood sugar control**. Activity causes muscles to burn sugar. Muscles will use the sugar in your bloodstream most readily as a form of energy and will ensure sugar in your blood won't be stored and converted to fat…

Dyna-Band® costs £10.50. Buy it from John Lewis, sports shops and www.dynaband.co.uk.

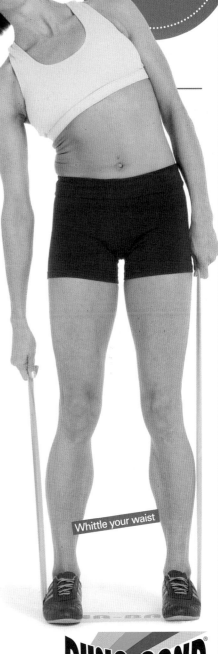

Whittle your waist

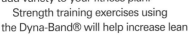

Tone your triceps

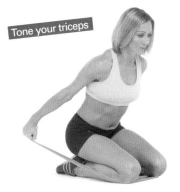

Trim your tummy

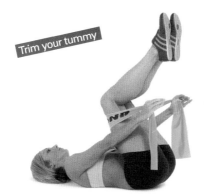

DYNA-BAND®
THE WORK-OUT THAT WORKS

ANTI-AGEING POWER CIRCUIT

This workout will take you just 30 minutes but is designed to work all parts of your body, including your bones. Try it three times weekly, alongside regular aerobic exercise. Throughout the circuit, focus on good form — make sure each move is high-quality to prevent injury and super-charge the benefits.

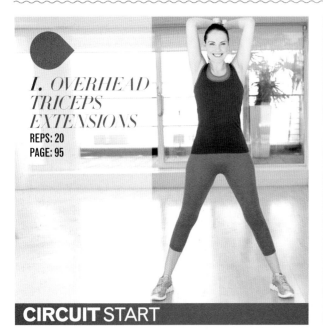

1. OVERHEAD TRICEPS EXTENSIONS
REPS: 20
PAGE: 95

CIRCUIT START

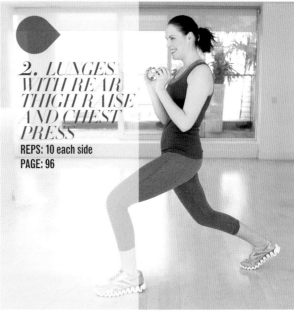

2. LUNGES WITH REAR THIGH RAISE AND CHEST PRESS
REPS: 10 each side
PAGE: 96

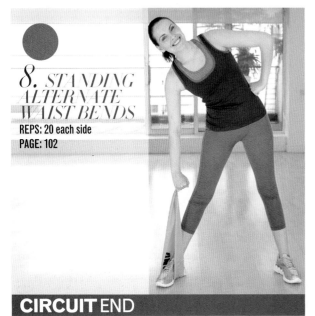

8. STANDING ALTERNATE WAIST BENDS
REPS: 20 each side
PAGE: 102

CIRCUIT END

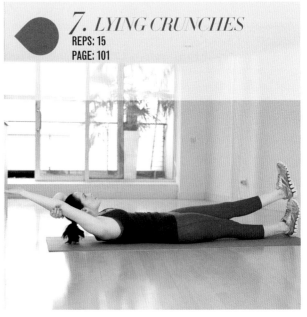

7. LYING CRUNCHES
REPS: 15
PAGE: 101

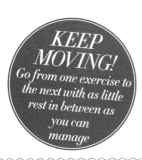

KEEP MOVING! Go from one exercise to the next with as little rest in between as you can manage

3. LYING DOWN OUTER THIGH EXERCISE
REPS: 10 each side
PAGE: 97

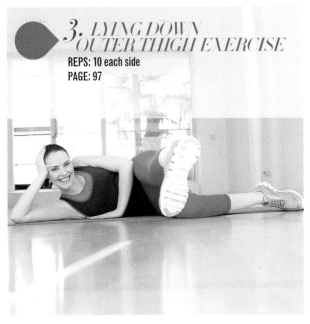

4. INNER THIGH RAISES
REPS: 10 each side
PAGE: 98

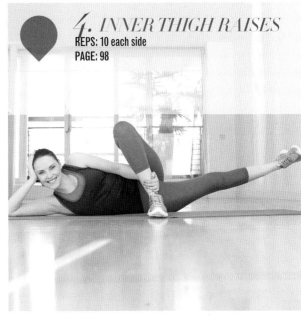

6. REAR THIGH RAISES
REPS: 10 each side
PAGE: 100

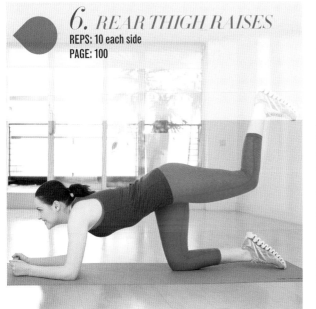

5. LYING DOWN SINGLE ARM CHEST FLYE
REPS: 10 each side
PAGE: 99

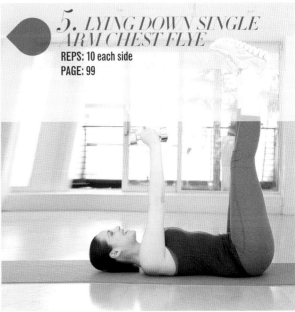

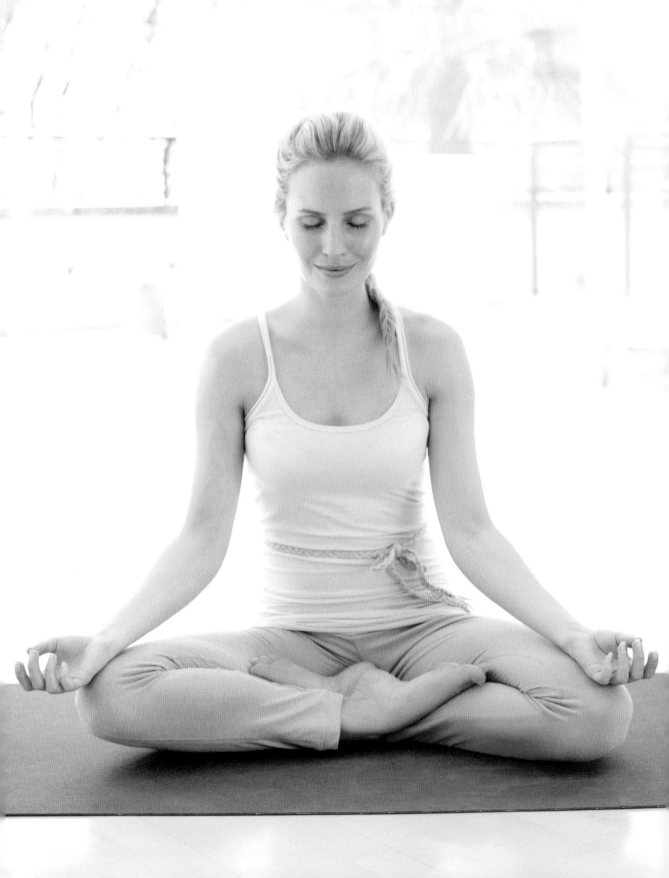

Your mind

It's not just how you treat your body that determines how fast you age. What's going on in your mind plays a big part too. The adage 'you're only as old as you feel' is true, say experts at Purdue University, US, who found people who view the ageing process with optimism and confidence are more likely to age gracefully. This chapter is about nourishing your mind and soul.

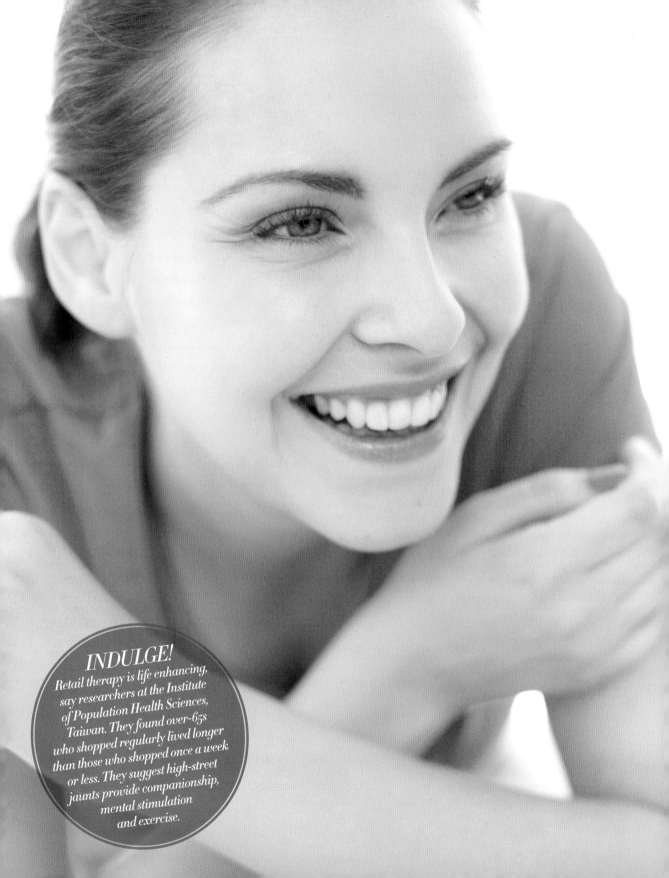

INDULGE!
Retail therapy is life enhancing, say researchers at the Institute of Population Health Sciences, Taiwan. They found over-65s who shopped regularly lived longer than those who shopped once a week or less. They suggest high-street jaunts provide companionship, mental stimulation and exercise.

Mind over matter

Ever feel older than you are? Think again! You can start shedding the years and feeling more vibrant just by changing your attitude to life

We all know someone whose youthful vitality belies their age. Equally, you're just as likely to have come across people who seem far older than their years. Attitude is everything in the ageing process; it's not just how you treat your body but the way you feel about yourself that than can keep you looking and feeling youthful. Positivity makes you resilient and, according to the latest research, can even have a positive impact on your body at a cellular level. It helps boost your immune system and also helps your body's systems regenerate.

Whether it's because optimism affects us on a biological level or simply encourages sound lifestyle habits, research repeatedly shows buoyant, sociable people are likely to stay healthier for longer. A recent review of more than 160 studies, published in *Applied Psychology: Health and Well-Being,* on the connection between a positive mental attitude and overall health and longevity has found clear evidence happier people enjoy a better sense of wellbeing and longer lives. Here's how to think yourself young.

NUTURE YOUR FRIENDSHIPS
According to research at Brigham Young University in Utah, being lonely can affect your health as adversely as smoking or a bad diet. But by friends, we mean real-life interaction rather through a computer screen; two studies at the University of Arizona have shown cyber relationships don't stave off feelings of loneliness.

LOVE WHAT YOU DO
Studies show that a satisfying work life enriches us, and this includes volunteer work. People who give their time for good causes are proven to have a lower mortality rate and be more physically able to cope with chronic pain or heart disease.

> 66 *Research shows buoyant, sociable people are likely to stay healthier for longer* 99

THINK YOURSELF LUCKY
Research by Professor Richard Wiseman at the University of Hertfordshire shows good luck is a state of mind – and we can maximise our chances of something good happening by creating, noticing and acting on opportunities and listening to our 'gut feelings'. When you're faced with a bad situation, turn it around by imaging how things could have been worse and considering practical solutions.

BE FEARLESS
Keep challenging yourself – take risks and get out of your comfort zone every once in a while to push your confidence levels sky-high. It could be as simple as talking to one stranger a day or as ambitious as changing your career and retraining, travelling to an exotic country or entering a marathon. Whatever it is, just make sure it really tests you! Remember, as we get older, we're more likely to regret the things we haven't done than the things we have.

HAPPY HUGS
Touch is the ultimate anti-ageing sense. Whether it's a hug, massage or holding hands, touch lowers the heart rate, eases pain and even affects our outlook on life. Researchers at Cedars-Sinai Hospital in LA found Swedish deep massage can trigger measurable changes in the body's immune function. Meanwhile, studies at Yale University show the feel of objects around us, even those we're sitting on, can affect our behaviour and thought patterns. The softer and more comforting they are, the more likely we are to feel positive. You can also boost your heart health by the simple act of hugging. A team from the University of North Carolina studied the effects of hugging in couples and found it ups levels of oxytocin, the bonding hormone, and reduces blood pressure. So when you feel stressed, reach out – literally.

De-stress, look younger!

Stress doesn't just leave you feeling frazzled. If you're not careful, it can take its toll on your looks and health too

A little bit of stress never did any harm – in fact, it can spur you into action, making you more productive and zippy. But from your digestion to your hair, your immunity to your heart, in abundance, stress can have tangible effects.

On a superficial level, stress triggers bad habits; you're less likely to eat well and may neglect exercise. But it also has biological effects. A University of California study found sustained periods of stress can add 10 years to the age of a woman's cells. It triggers rushes of a hormone called cortisol, which encourages fat to be laid down around the abdomen, and is detrimental to bone health. Plus, cortisol can accelerate skin ageing – your skin's defence system goes into overdrive, causing inflammation, which can weaken collagen structure, leading to sagginess. According to dermatologists, just two to three months of stress could damage skin and lead to wrinkles. It can also trigger other skin problems, such as acne and eczema.

The odd stressful day probably won't do your looks much harm, but a few-angst-filled weeks or months could take their toll. Here's how to take control.

UNDERSTAND YOUR MIND

Whether or not you feel stressed comes down to how you perceive a situation rather than what's actually going on. For instance, you might feel terrified at the thought of doing a presentation and lose sleep for weeks beforehand, while a

> ❝ *Make a point of de-stressing daily, whether it's a walk in the park or a yoga class* ❞

colleague will relish the challenge. Being aware of your natural predisposition and what spurs your anxieties is the first step to getting a handle on them. Step back and examine why you find particular situations angst-inducing.

IDENTIFY YOUR PRESSURE PATTERNS

We all have our own repetitive thought patterns – a set way of thinking when we face stressful situations. If you have a need for approval, for example, you'll measure your worth according to what others think of you and feel anxious if you assume you're not up to scratch. If you're

a 'catastrophiser', you'll always believe the worst and jump to conclusions, even if you have no evidence to back up your view. Identify and deconstruct your habitual way of approaching issues – and ask, is there a healthier alternative?

BECOME STRESS-HARDY

In the midst of a crisis, it can be hard to motivate yourself to do the very things that can help you feel better. Identify your 'back-up' plan – people, activities or commitments that have, in the past, helped you deal better with stress and feel less isolated. Do you have a friend whose energy is infectious? Or do you have a favourite walk that lifts your spirits? Think ahead about the tools you can use in an emergency.

SMALL CHANGES

To prevent long-term accumulation of anxiety, make a point of de-stressing daily, whether it's a walk in the park, deep breathing or an evening yoga class. Always take a break from your desk, even if it's only for 10 minutes, and avoid skipping meals. Watch your posture and body language – smile and laugh as much as you can; research shows it can have a positive effect on your health.

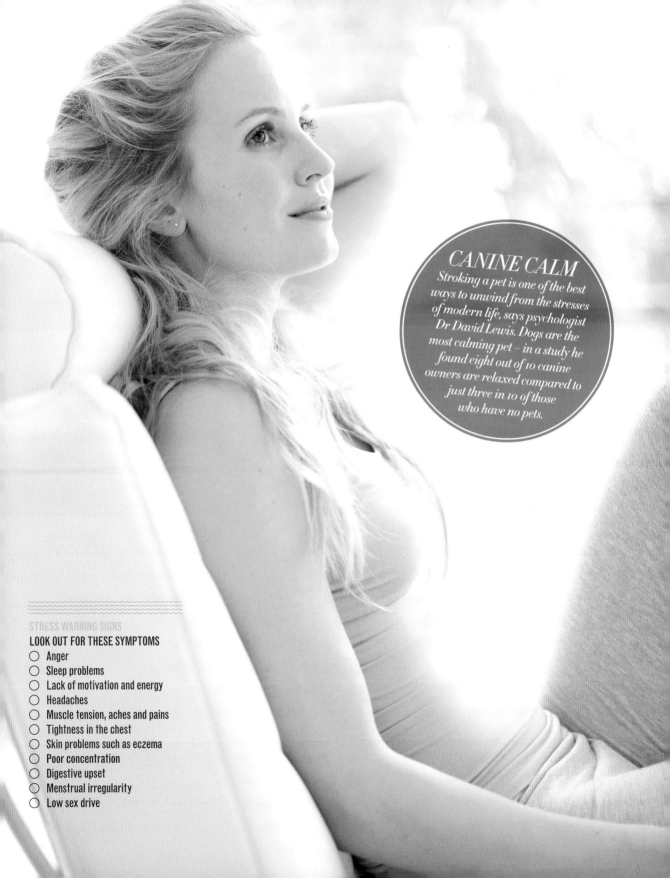

CANINE CALM
Stroking a pet is one of the best ways to unwind from the stresses of modern life, says psychologist Dr David Lewis. Dogs are the most calming pet – in a study he found eight out of 10 canine owners are relaxed compared to just three in 10 of those who have no pets.

STRESS WARNING SIGNS
LOOK OUT FOR THESE SYMPTOMS
- Anger
- Sleep problems
- Lack of motivation and energy
- Headaches
- Muscle tension, aches and pains
- Tightness in the chest
- Skin problems such as eczema
- Poor concentration
- Digestive upset
- Menstrual irregularity
- Low sex drive

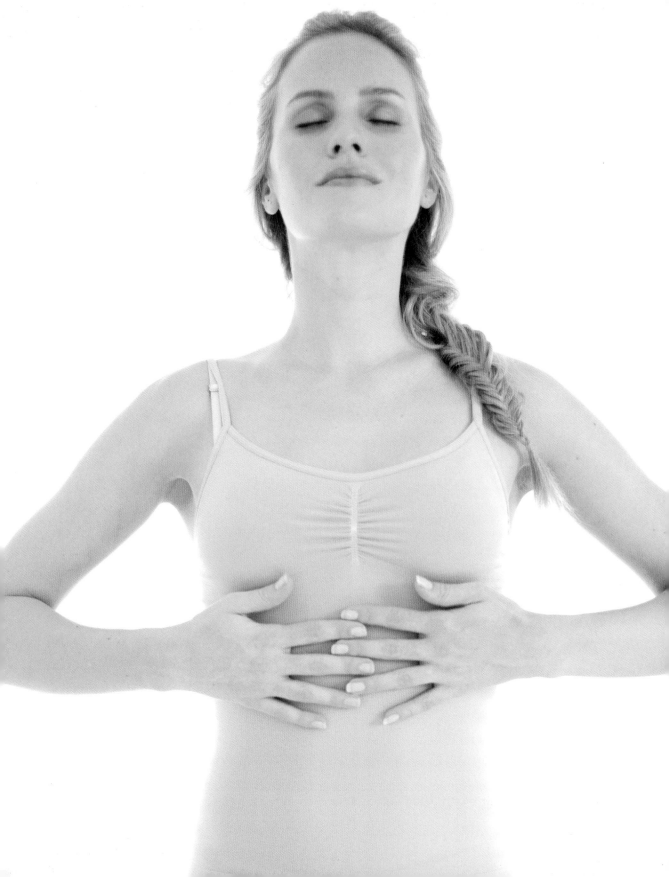

Breathe yourself better

Balance your active life with plenty of chill-out time.
Breathing well paves the way to a younger body

We breathe so instinctively – more than 23,000 times a day, in fact – that most of us have forgotten how to do it properly and take our lungs for granted. But using the full might of your lungs can bestow age-defying benefits, including increased levels of confidence, energy and calm – and, studies show, lower blood pressure. This all helps to keep the wrinkles at bay. We're hard-wired from birth to breathe deeply and use our full lung capacity, engaging the diaphragm and intercostal muscles (between the ribs), but, over time, our breath tends to become shallower. Breathing poorly results in low energy levels and poorly nourished cells. Stress is partly to blame – and it's a vicious circle because restricted breathing increases anxiety further. Here's how to breathe yourself younger.

Mindful breathing

○ Re-teach yourself how to breathe from your belly not your chest; pushing out your lower abdomen gently while inhaling and returning it on the exhale. Also, concentrate on breathing through your nose, rather than your mouth, as it acts as an air filter.

Breathing poorly results in low energy levels and poorly nourished cells. Stress is partly to blame

○ Breathe in and out of your feet, figuratively speaking. On an out breath, visualise roots growing down from your feet and into the floor – this helps ground you and slow down racing thoughts. Remove obvious physical tension in your body by shrugging your shoulders, and uncrossing arms and legs.

○ Breathe in stages. Imagine your abdomen is made up of different parts and inhale from your lower abdomen to your chest for a count of four. Then exhale from your nose to the count of nine. Breathing out for longer than you breathe in helps trigger your body's relaxation mechanism.

○ Spot check your breathing patterns throughout the day, but also devote some time to looking after your lungs, particularly if you're prone to stress. T'ai chi and yoga focus on breathing and have added fitness benefits. Try meditation too; research published in the *Journal of Neuroscience* shows those who practised meditation for a five-year period had a biological age of around 12 years younger than their real age.

BOOST YOUR LUNG POWER...
Your lung capacity declines dramatically by the time you reach your 70s, as your respiratory muscles lose strength, your rib cage becomes less flexible and the alveoli, the tiny grape-like sacs of your lungs, start to thin and become less efficient at processing oxygen and carbon dioxide. You can protect your lungs and maximise your breathing from a young age by not smoking, taking plenty of aerobic exercise and wearing a mask if you're doing DIY or exposed to fumes and vapours.

Get your beauty sleep!

We've all heard the benefits of having enough sleep.
Here's how to ensure you get a good night's rest

It's not called beauty sleep for nothing. Sleep is essential for beautiful, glowing skin and helping your body stay at its peak. When you sleep, your body produces growth hormone, vital for cell renewal. We've all noticed the dull skin and hollow eyes we get after a bad night's sleep. A study at Karolinska Institute in Stockholm found chronically sleep-deprived people appear less attractive and unhealthier than those who are well rested. Lack of sleep not only weakens the immune system, it's implicated in a variety of conditions including heart disease, stroke, diabetes and depression; none of which will help you feel youthful! To stay looking and feeling energised and youthful, you need to aim for a regular, set amount of good-quality shut-eye. Here's how to do it.

HOW MUCH IS ENOUGH?

Don't get hung up on how much sleep you need – it's all about quality, not quantity. Everyone's different (average sleep time varies from six to eight or more hours), so listen to your body and work out the optimum amount of time you feel you should sleep for.

GET INTO A ROUTINE

Maintain regular sleeping times, even at weekends, to send strong messages to your body clock and wean it off alarms. Make sure you get a 10-minute dose of direct daylight in the morning to help set your body clock.

> *Sleep is about quality not quantity and everyone's different, so listen to your body*

HAVE A NAP

If you're a good sleeper, and it's practical, take a recharging cat-nap during the natural afternoon slump. But don't snooze for longer than 20 minutes or you'll enter deep sleep and feel worse afterwards.

CREATE A RESTFUL SPACE

Ensure your boudoir is conducive to sleep. Get a good-quality mattress and bedding, keep your laptop and TV out, declutter, darken and cool the space – the optimal temperature is from 16°C to 18°C.

WIND DOWN BEFORE BED

Avoid pre-slumber stimulants, such as scary films, high-impact exercise, caffeine, alcohol and heavy meals (sex is fine, as it's also relaxing). Try some wind-down tools to help beat insomnia, including meditation, a warm bath, a warm, milky drink or camomile tea and an undemanding paperback. Spritz your pillow with a calming aromatherapy blend that includes lavender and empty your mind of stressful thoughts – have a notebook beside your bed and note down a to-do list for the next day if necessary.

LIGHTS OUT

If you find it hard to nod off, invest in some blackout curtains to block out street lights. Keep your home lighting soft as you wind down for bed and always switch off any light sources before you hit the pillow.

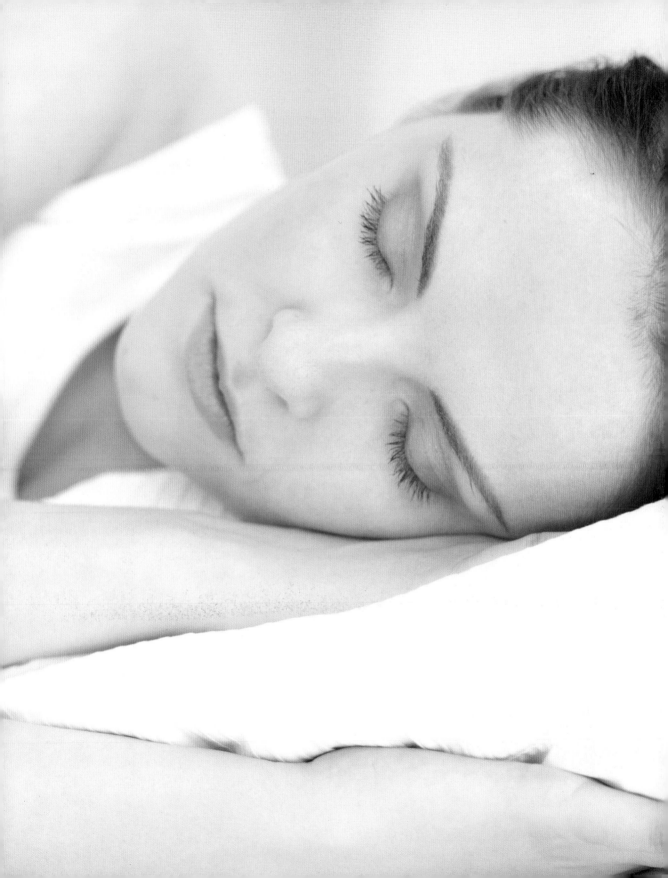

Youthful yoga

We've picked the best age- and gravity-defying yoga poses
to help you look young and stay super flexible

Yoga essentials

Yoga is pretty kit-light and most classes will provide equipment, but these are the common props you'll encounter in classes.

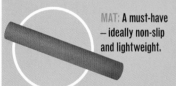

MAT: A must-have – ideally non-slip and lightweight.

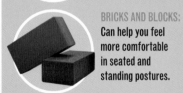

BRICKS AND BLOCKS: Can help you feel more comfortable in seated and standing postures.

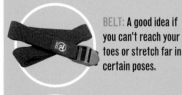

BELT: A good idea if you can't reach your toes or stretch far in certain poses.

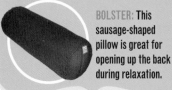

BOLSTER: This sausage-shaped pillow is great for opening up the back during relaxation.

We're all familiar with the stress-busting, body-shaping benefits of yoga, but studies show it can also protect your body from age-associated illnesses. Following a regular yoga practise can help reduce the body's inflammation response, implicated in arthritis, heart disease and stroke, among other illnesses. You can find a handful of our favourite anti-ageing poses on the following pages.

> **Studies show regular yoga practice can protect your body from age-associated illness**

FIND YOUR STYLE

Confused by the multitude of yoga styles out there? Although there are bedrock postures, the speed and intensity of classes varies greatly. If you're a novice, even if you consider yourself to be very fit, start with a gentle form, such as hatha or Iyengar. These are the common types:

IYENGAR Slow and precise, this style encourages you to use accessories such as belts to aid postures.

HATHA is an umbrella form so classes tend to include a mix of asanas, breathing exercises and meditation and go at a managable pace.

ASHTANGA Gymnastic and speedy so it has an aerobic element. Classes comprise of a precise set of asanas that flow together, so you're rarely still.

BIKRAM 26 traditional asanas, perfomed quickly and in a very hot room. Definitely not for novice yogis!

KUNDALINI An expressive form focusing on meditation, chanting and breathing.

Before you begin...

○ Wait four to five hours after a heavy meal, around two hours after a snack.
○ Practise in loose fitting clothes and bare feet.
○ Always work on a non-slip mat. Use blocks, bolsters and belts to assist your practice, where appropriate.
○ Although you should feel challenged during the poses, you shouldn't be in any pain. Ease yourself into them.
○ Breathe slowly and calmly, inhaling and exhaling through your nose.
○ Avoid inverted poses when you're menstruating, have or are recovering from head and neck injuries, have glaucoma or high blood pressure.

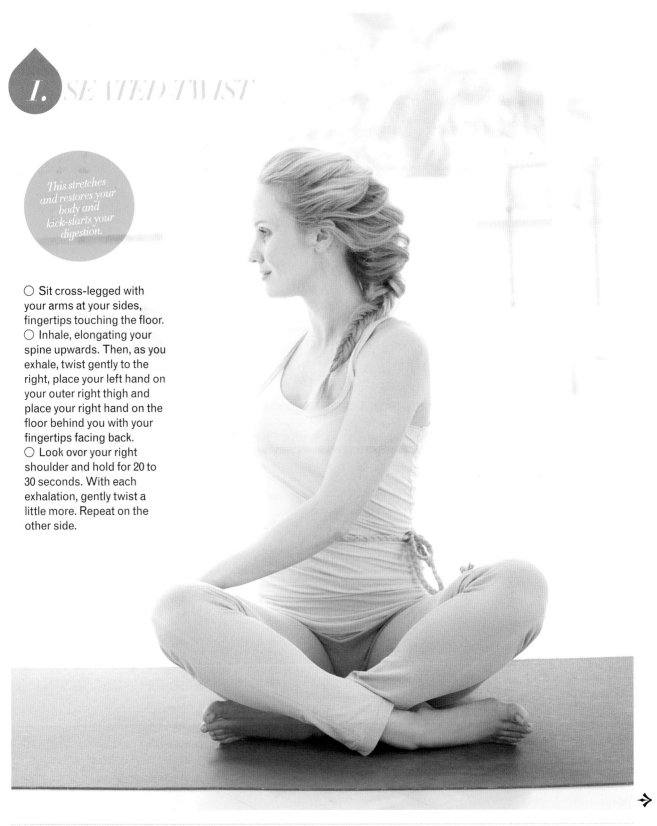

1. SEATED TWIST

This stretches and restores your body and kick-starts your digestion.

○ Sit cross-legged with your arms at your sides, fingertips touching the floor.
○ Inhale, elongating your spine upwards. Then, as you exhale, twist gently to the right, place your left hand on your outer right thigh and place your right hand on the floor behind you with your fingertips facing back.
○ Look ovor your right shoulder and hold for 20 to 30 seconds. With each exhalation, gently twist a little more. Repeat on the other side.

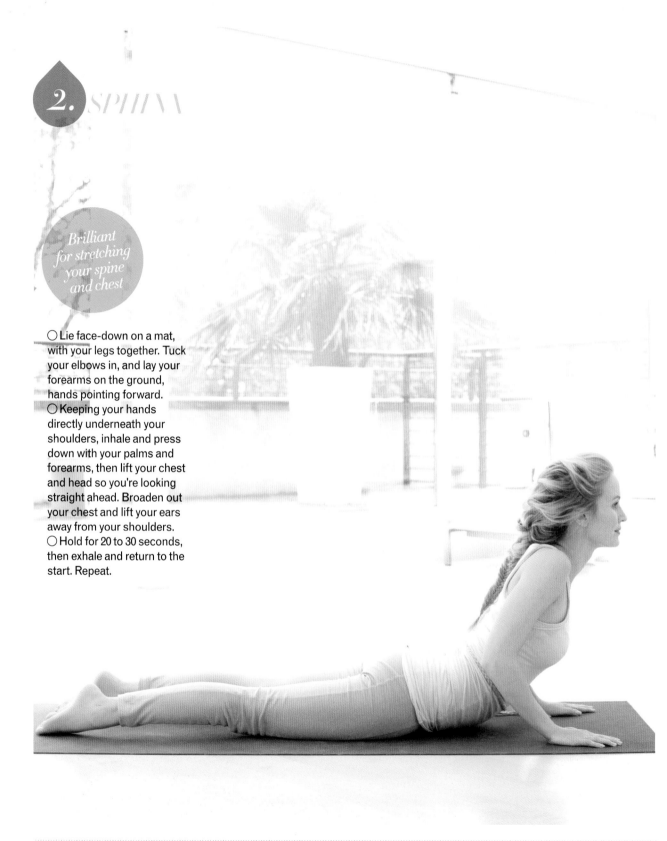

2. *SPHINX*

Brilliant for stretching your spine and chest

○ Lie face-down on a mat, with your legs together. Tuck your elbows in, and lay your forearms on the ground, hands pointing forward.

○ Keeping your hands directly underneath your shoulders, inhale and press down with your palms and forearms, then lift your chest and head so you're looking straight ahead. Broaden out your chest and lift your ears away from your shoulders.

○ Hold for 20 to 30 seconds, then exhale and return to the start. Repeat.

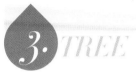

3. TREE

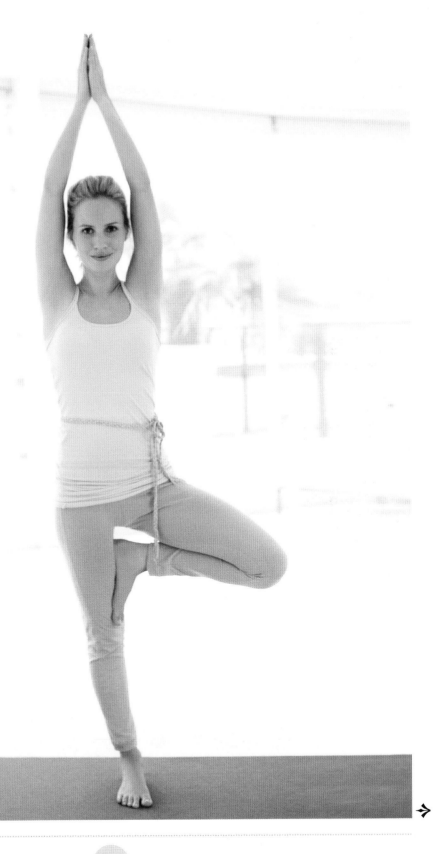

Builds strength in your feet, legs, bum and core muscles

○ Stand with your feet together. Moving your bodyweight onto your right foot, catch your left ankle and place the sole of your left foot on the inside of your right thigh. If that's too challenging, place it on your calf, but avoid your knee joint altogether.

○ Place your hands in prayer position in front of your chest and look straight ahead.

○ Hold, then inhale and extend your arms overhead, palms facing each other. Join your palms, without bending the elbows. Hold for 20 to 30 seconds, and repeat on the other leg.

4. DOWNWARD DOG

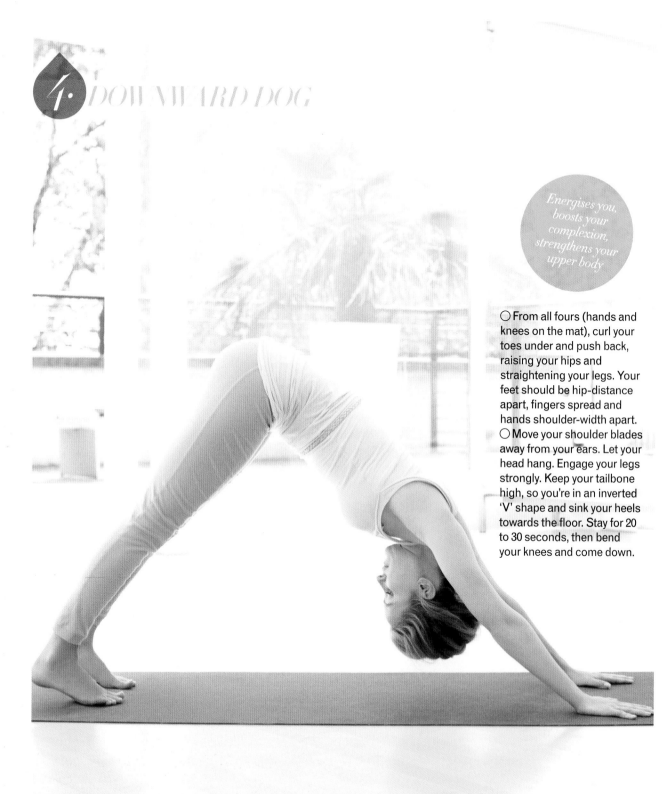

Energises you, boosts your complexion, strengthens your upper body

○ From all fours (hands and knees on the mat), curl your toes under and push back, raising your hips and straightening your legs. Your feet should be hip-distance apart, fingers spread and hands shoulder-width apart.

○ Move your shoulder blades away from your ears. Let your head hang. Engage your legs strongly. Keep your tailbone high, so you're in an inverted 'V' shape and sink your heels towards the floor. Stay for 20 to 30 seconds, then bend your knees and come down.

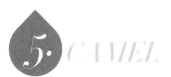

5. CAMEL

Stretches your upper body. Builds flexibility in your spine. Boosts your digestive and reproductive systems

○ Kneel on the floor with knees and feet parallel and hip-width apart, pressing your shins and the tops of your feet onto the floor. Rest your hands on your hips and gently arch your back, moving your tail bone forward, but keeping thighs perpendicular. Move slowly.

○ When you're ready, reach down and place your right palm on your right foot. If this is enough for you, stay here then come up and repeat on the left. Or, if you feel comfortable, place both hands down at the same time.

○ Keep your neck in a neutral position or drop your head back. Stretch open your chest. If you can't touch your feet without compressing your lower back, turn your toes under to lift your heels. Stay here for 30 seconds to a minute.

○ To release, place your hands on your hips, inhale and lift your head and chest, leading with your heart.

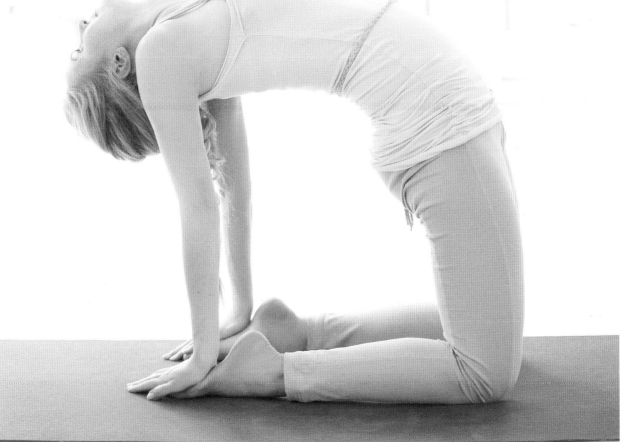

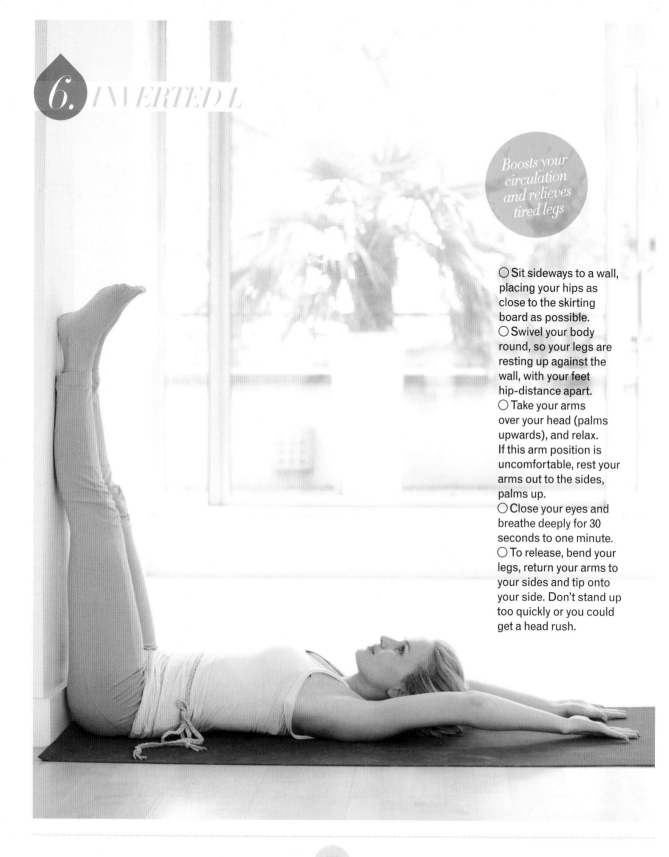

6. INVERTED L

◯ Sit sideways to a wall, placing your hips as close to the skirting board as possible.
◯ Swivel your body round, so your legs are resting up against the wall, with your feet hip-distance apart.
◯ Take your arms over your head (palms upwards), and relax. If this arm position is uncomfortable, rest your arms out to the sides, palms up.
◯ Close your eyes and breathe deeply for 30 seconds to one minute.
◯ To release, bend your legs, return your arms to your sides and tip onto your side. Don't stand up too quickly or you could get a head rush.

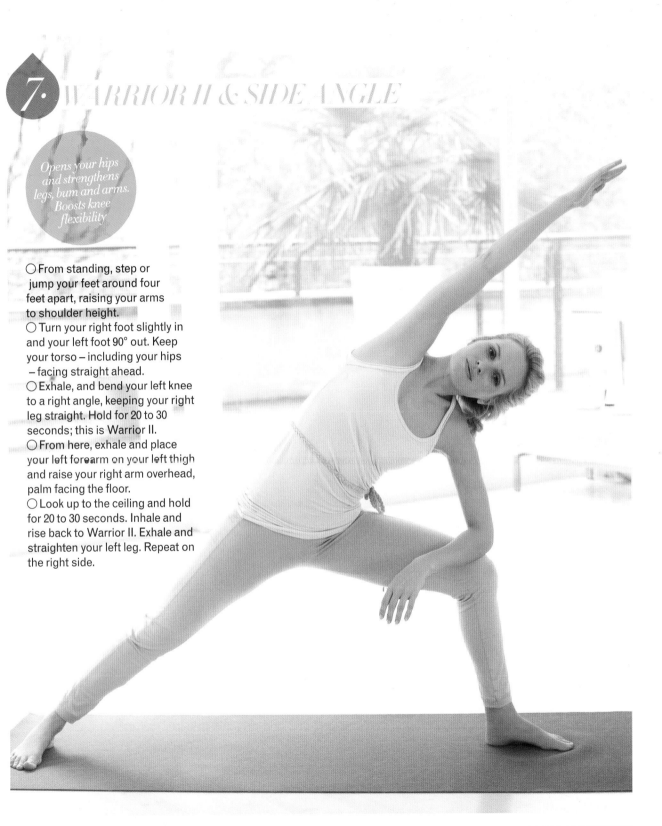

7. WARRIOR II & SIDE ANGLE

Opens your hips and strengthens legs, bum and arms. Boosts knee flexibility

○ From standing, step or jump your feet around four feet apart, raising your arms to shoulder height.

○ Turn your right foot slightly in and your left foot 90° out. Keep your torso – including your hips – facing straight ahead.

○ Exhale, and bend your left knee to a right angle, keeping your right leg straight. Hold for 20 to 30 seconds; this is Warrior II.

○ From here, exhale and place your left forearm on your left thigh and raise your right arm overhead, palm facing the floor.

○ Look up to the ceiling and hold for 20 to 30 seconds. Inhale and rise back to Warrior II. Exhale and straighten your left leg. Repeat on the right side.

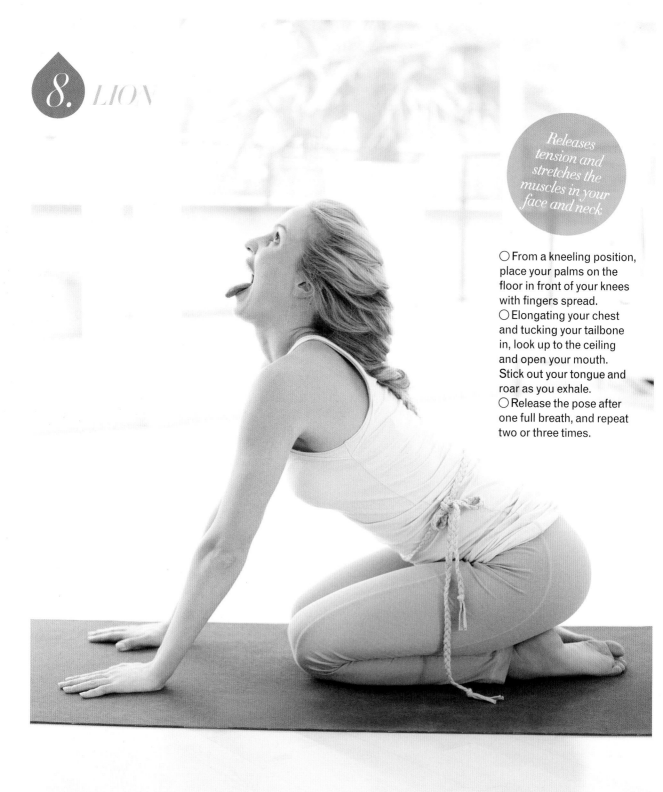

8. LION

Releases tension and stretches the muscles in your face and neck

○ From a kneeling position, place your palms on the floor in front of your knees with fingers spread.

○ Elongating your chest and tucking your tailbone in, look up to the ceiling and open your mouth. Stick out your tongue and roar as you exhale.

○ Release the pose after one full breath, and repeat two or three times.

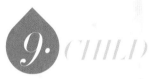

9. CHILD

Eases out your neck and back and calms your mind

○ Sit on your heels with your knees apart and big toes touching.
○ Inhale, then, as you exhale, bring your forehead to the floor and let your arms rest by your sides, palms facing the ceiling.
○ Relax here for as long as you like, breathing gently.

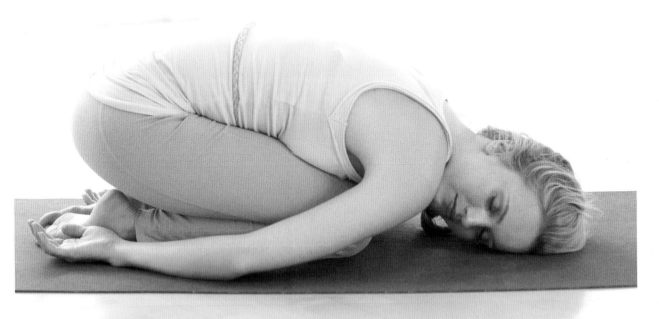

Directory

Beauty – skincare, bodycare and cosmetics

AETERNA
www.highernature.co.uk

AROMATHERAPY ASSOCIATES
020 8569 7030
www.aromatherapy
associates.com

AVEDA
0800 054 2979
www.aveda.co.uk

BARE ESCENTUALS
0870 850 6655
www.bareescentuals.co.uk

BAREFOOT BOTANICALS
0870 220 2273
www.barefoot-
botanicals.com

THE BODY SHOP
0800 0929090
www.thebodyshop.co.uk

CLARINS
uk.clarins.com

COMVITA
www.comvita.co.uk

DR HAUSCHKA
01386 791022
www.drhauschka.co.uk

DERMALOGICA
www.dermalogica.com/uk/

DERMA E
www.dermae.net

ELEMIS
01278 727830
www.elemis.co.uk

ESPA
01252 742800
www.espaonline.com

ESSENTIAL CARE
01638 716593
www.essential-care.co.uk

ESTÉE LAUDER
0800 054 2444
www.esteelauder.co.uk

EURECIN
www.eurecin.co.uk

GOODSKIN LABS
0870 034 2663
www.goodskinlabs.co.uk

GREEN PEOPLE
01403 740350
www.greenpeople.co.uk

ILA SPA
01608 677676
www.ila-spa.com

INLIGHT
www.inlight-online.co.uk

INIKA
020 7494 4571
www.inikacosmetics.co.uk

JASON
www.jason
naturalcare.co.uk

JURLIQUE
020 3205 3845
www.jurlique.co.uk

LAVERA
01557 870266
www.lavera.co.uk

LAURA MERCIER
www.lauramercier.com

LIVING NATURE
0845 250 8455
www.livingnature.com

LIZ EARLE NATURALLY ACTIVE SKINCARE
01983 813913
www.lizearle.com

LOVE LULA
www.lovelula.com

MÁDARA
01557 870266
www.pravera.co.uk

MARGARET DABBS
www.margaretdabbs.co.uk

MD FORMULATIONS
www.bareescentuals.co.uk

NEAL'S YARD REMEDIES
01747 834600
www.nealsyardremedies.com

NIP + FAB
020 7351 1720
www.nipandfab.com

DR NICK LOWE
020 7499 3223
www.drnicklowe.com

NOVOSTRATA
0845 004 8473
www.novostrata.co.uk

NUDE SKINCARE
0800 634 4366
www.nudeskincare.com

L'OCCITANE
020 7907 0301
www.loccitane.com

OLE HENRIKSEN
www.olehenriksen.com

THE ORGANIC PHARMACY
0844 800 8399
www.theorganicpharmacy.com

ORGANIC SURGE
01955 606061
www.organicsurge.com

ORIGINS
0800 054 2888
www.origins.co.uk

OSKIA SKINCARE
020 7978 0207
www.oskiaskincare.com

PALMER'S
COCOA FORMULA
www.uk.palmers.com

PERRICONE
0800 917 8698
www.perriconemd.co.uk

REN
020 7724 2900
www.renskincare.com

THE SANCTUARY
0844 875 8443
www.thesanctuary.co.uk

SHIFFA
www.shiffa.com

SPIEZIA
0870 850 8851
www.spieziaorganics.com

THIS WORKS
020 8543 3544
www.thisworks.com

TRILOGY
www.trilogyproducts.com

VAISHALY
www.vaishaly.com

WELEDA
0115 944 8222
www.weleda.co.uk

YES TO CARROTS
www.yestocarrots.com

Hair

BUMBLE & BUMBLE
0800 014 7424
www.bumbleand
bumble.com

EVOLVE
0844 991 0061
www.evolvebeauty.co.uk

DANIEL FIELD
0800 077 8270
www.danielfield.com

JOHN MASTERS
www.johnmasters.co.uk

KEVIN MURPHY
01179 270434
www.kevinmurphystore.com

MOP
01179 270432
www.mophair.com

PHYTO
www.phyto.com/en/

SCHWARZKOPF
01296 314000
www.schwarzkopf.co.uk

TRESEMME
www.tresemme.com

Health and fitness

ASICS
www.asics.co.uk

BRITISH
ACUPUNCTURE
COUNCIL
www.acupuncture.org.uk

BRITISH
ASSOCIATION OF
DERMATOLOGISTS
www.bad.org.uk

BRITISH DENTAL
ASSOCIATION
www.bdasmile.org

BRITISH SWIMMING
www.swimming.org

BRITISH WHEEL
OF YOGA
www.bwy.org.uk

COMVITA
01628 779460
www.comvita.co.uk

CTC – UK'S
NATIONAL CYCLISTS'
ORGANISATION
www.ctc.org.uk

DYNA-BAND
0845 305 4131
www.dynaband.co.uk

ENERGY BODIES
0871 903 0000
www.energybodies.co.uk

EVA FRASER
020 7937 6616
www.evafraser.com

FACE YOGA
www.yogaface.net

HEALTH SPAN
0800 731 2377
www.healthspan.co.uk

METHOD PUTKISTO
www.methodputkisto.com

NIFTY
www.theniftyfacelift.co.uk

NIKE WOMEN
store.nike.com/UK

PILATES FOUNDATION
www.pilatesfoundation.com

PUKKA
0845 375 1744
www.pukkaherbs.com

RAMBLERS'
ASSOCIATION
www.ramblers.org.uk

➔

REGISTER OF EXERCISE PROFESSIONALS
www.exerciseregister.org

SHOCK ABSORBER
0500 362430
www.shockabsorber.co.uk

SLENDERTONE FACE
www.slendertoneface.com

SO ORGANIC
www.soorganic.com

SUN SMART
www.sunsmart.org.uk

TAI CHI UNION FOR GREAT BRITAIN
www.taichiunion.com

TISSERAND
www.tisserand.com

THE SOIL ASSOCIATION
www.soilassociation.org

TUA TREND BY TINA RICHARDS
www.tuatrendface.com

DR ANDREW WEIL
www.drweil.com

YOGA MATTERS
020 8888 8588
www.yogamatters.com

ZUMBA
www.zumba.com

Diet and supplements

BIOCARE
www.biocare.co.uk

CENTRUM
www.centrum.com

EFAMOL
01372 379828
www.efamol.com

HEALTHSPAN
www.healthspan.co.uk

HIGHER NATURE
0800 458 4747
www.highernature.co.uk

IMEDEEN
0845 555 4499
www.imedeen.co.uk

KINETIC
0845 072 5825
www.kinetic4health.co.uk

NATURE'S BEST
01892 552117
www.naturesbest.co.uk

PROTO-COL
0844 811 2906
www.proto-col.com

PURE XP
020 7738 3399
www.pure-xp.com

REFLEX
01273 711616
www.reflex-nutrition.com

SALUS
01925 825679
www.salusuk.com

SOLGAR
01782 634744
www.solgar.co.uk

SUN CHLORELLA
0800 008 6166
www.sunchlorella.co.uk

UDO'S CHOICE
www.udoschoice.co.uk

VEGA VITAMINS & HERBALS
08452 267300
www.vegavitamins.co.uk

VIRIDIAN
01327 878050
www.viridian-nutrition.com

VITABIOTICS
www.vitabiotics.com

Treatments

ANNEE DE MAMIEL
www.demamiel.com

BLISS
020 7590 6146
www.blissworld.co.uk

CACI
020 8731 5678
www.caci-international.co.uk

CRYSTAL CLEAR
0151 709 7227
www.crystalclear.co.uk

ELEMIS
01278 727830
www.elemis.co.uk

EMMA HARDIE
020 7629 6969
www.emmahardie.com

ENERGY BODIES
www.energybodies.co.uk

GUINOT
uk.guinot.com

KARIN HERZOG
0800 056 2428
www.karinherzog.co.uk

ORALIFT
www.oralift.com

RANI MIRZA
020 7589 9080
www.ranimirza.co.uk

SPECIAL OFFER!
TRY 3 ISSUES FOR JUST £1

3 ISSUES FOR £1

Keep up-to-date with the latest trends in health, fitness and nutrition, and maintain your motivation by having news, in-depth features and expert tips delivered to your door every month!

SUBSCRIBE TODAY & RECEIVE:

✔ Your first **3 issues for £1**
✔ **22% saving** on all subsequent issues
✔ **FREE delivery** direct to your door
✔ **Expert advice** on health, fitness and nutrition every month!

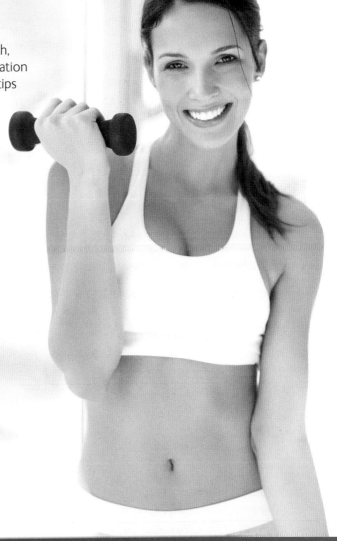

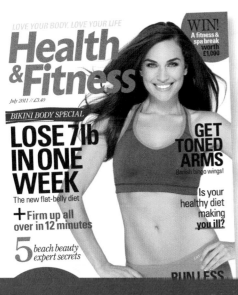

Order online at **www.dennismags.co.uk/healthandfitness** or
CALL 0844 499 1763
using offer code: **G1108LY**

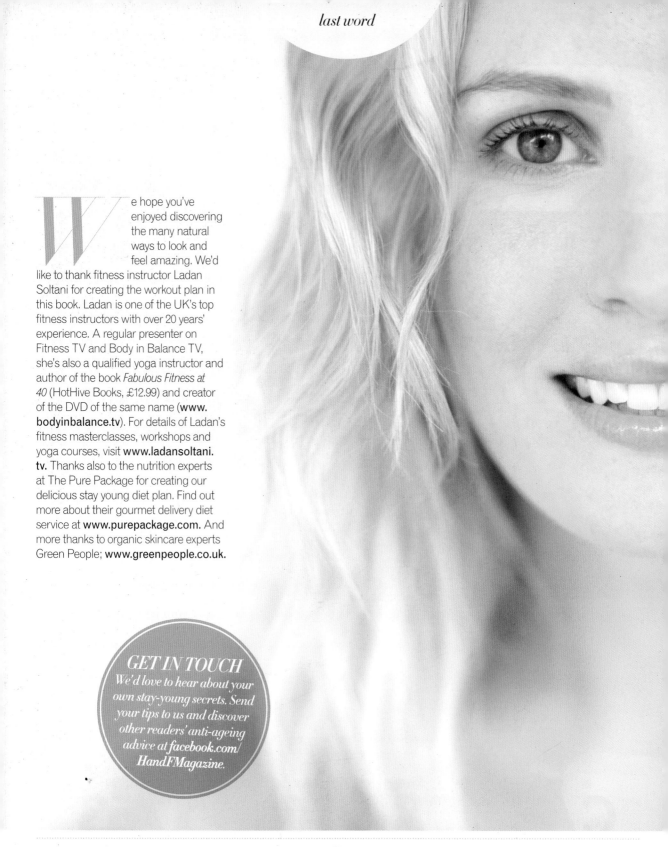

We hope you've enjoyed discovering the many natural ways to look and feel amazing. We'd like to thank fitness instructor Ladan Soltani for creating the workout plan in this book. Ladan is one of the UK's top fitness instructors with over 20 years' experience. A regular presenter on Fitness TV and Body in Balance TV, she's also a qualified yoga instructor and author of the book *Fabulous Fitness at 40* (HotHive Books, £12.99) and creator of the DVD of the same name (**www.bodyinbalance.tv**). For details of Ladan's fitness masterclasses, workshops and yoga courses, visit **www.ladansoltani.tv**. Thanks also to the nutrition experts at The Pure Package for creating our delicious stay young diet plan. Find out more about their gourmet delivery diet service at **www.purepackage.com**. And more thanks to organic skincare experts Green People; **www.greenpeople.co.uk**.

GET IN TOUCH
We'd love to hear about your own stay-young secrets. Send your tips to us and discover other readers' anti-ageing advice at facebook.com/HandFMagazine.